THE NATURE OF INCLUSIVE PLAY

This book provides designers, planners, educators, and therapists with the practical information required to remove inequity in outdoor spaces, by creating inviting and inclusive solutions so that all children and their families, regardless of situation or circumstance, can experience the joys and benefits of outdoor play without stigma.

It is the first of its kind, co-written by an occupational therapist and landscape architect both with proven expertise in inclusive play space design. *The Nature of Inclusive Play* fills an untapped niche in promoting the value of outdoor play. It focuses on what embodies play and shows how, through inclusive outdoor play design, developmental skills can be enriched. The topics covered in the book include:

- a discussion of the health benefits associated with being outdoors
- the history of and value of play
- an overview of typical child development
- the importance of sensory regulation
- an inclusive design review process
- design guidelines.

All topics are supplemented with nine applicable case studies of inclusive outdoor play spaces with features that reflect inclusive[+] principles, including examples from North America and Africa. It is a much-needed guide for landscape architects, urban planners, allied health care professionals, early childhood educators, academics, and students.

Amy Wagenfeld, PhD, OTR/L, SCEM, EDAC, FAOTA, is an occupational therapist, therapeutic and universal design consultant, educator, researcher, and author. She is an Affiliate Associate Professor in the University of Washington's

Department of Landscape Architecture and is the Principal of Amy Wagenfeld | Design, a therapeutic design consulting organization. Amy is a Fellow of the American Occupational Therapy Association, holds evidence-based design accreditation and certification (EDAC) through the Center for Health Design, specialty certification in environmental modifications (SCEM) through the American Occupational Therapy Association, and certification in Healthcare Garden Design through the Chicago Botanical Garden. She was recently awarded the American Society of Landscape Architects Outstanding Service Award and the American Occupational Therapy Association Recognition of Achievement for her unique blending of occupational therapy and therapeutic design. Amy publishes and presents widely on topics related to nature and health and is co-author of the award-winning book *Therapeutic Gardens: Design for Healing Spaces* published by Timber Press and *Nature-Based Allied Health Practice* by Jessica Kingsley Publishers.

Chad Kennedy, PLA, CPSI, is a Principal Landscape Architect for a private design firm, O'Dell Engineering. He holds a master's degree in landscape architecture from Utah State University. His interest in design-oriented childhood development and psychologically healthy play environments originates from a yearlong interdisciplinary disability course he participated in at the Center for Persons with Disabilities at Utah State University nearly 20 years ago. Chad's experience there made a lasting impression, guiding his passion for creating outdoor environments that are sensitive to all forms of children's development needs, promote wellness and completeness, and provide unimpeded access to all who wish to participate. Chad has published numerous articles on child-focused design and presents nationally on these and related subjects. Under his direction as a partner, O'Dell Engineering has focused on designing health care gardens and recreational environments that meet those criteria, including many socially inclusive and sensory-integrated playgrounds.

THE NATURE OF INCLUSIVE PLAY

A Guide for Designers, Educators, and Therapists

Amy Wagenfeld and Chad Kennedy

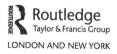

Routledge
Taylor & Francis Group

LONDON AND NEW YORK

Designed cover image: © Getty

First published 2024
by Routledge
4 Park Square, Milton Park, Abingdon, Oxon OX14 4RN

and by Routledge
605 Third Avenue, New York, NY 10158

Routledge is an imprint of the Taylor & Francis Group, an informa business

British Library Cataloguing-in-Publication Data
A catalogue record for this book is available from the British Library

Library of Congress Cataloging-in-Publication Data
Names: Wagenfeld, Amy, author. | Kennedy, Chad, author.
Title: The nature of inclusive play : a guide for designers, educators, and
therapists / Amy Wagenfeld and Chad Kennedy.
Description: Abingdon, Oxon ; New York, NY : Routledge, 2024. | Includes
bibliographical references and index.
Identifiers: LCCN 2023028528 (print) | LCCN 2023028529 (ebook) |
ISBN 9781032046020 (hardback) | ISBN 9781032045801 (paperback) |
ISBN 9781003193890 (ebook)
Subjects: LCSH: Play environments—Design and construction. | Outdoor
recreation for children. | Play—Social aspects. | Barrier-free design.
Classification: LCC GV425 .W34 2024 (print) | LCC GV425 (ebook) |
DDC 796.5083—dc23/eng/20230817
LC record available at https://lccn.loc.gov/2023028528
LC ebook record available at https://lccn.loc.gov/2023028529

ISBN: 978-1-032-04602-0 (hbk)
ISBN: 978-1-032-04580-1 (pbk)
ISBN: 978-1-003-19389-0 (ebk)

DOI: 10.4324/9781003193890

Typeset in TimesNewRoman
by codeMantra

For all children, past, present, and future.

CONTENTS

ACKNOWLEDGMENTS

I would like to thank the landscape architects and designers who welcomed me into their amazing world and invited me to work with them on design projects. It has been a lifetime dream come true, and having the opportunity to help create outdoor spaces that enable all children to flourish has been and continues to be profoundly meaningful. For my husband, Jeffrey Hsi, my gratitude runs deep for your unending support. For our son, David Hsi, whom I had the privilege of helping to nurture a lifelong love of play, you are an inspiration. I love you both dearly.

Amy

I express gratitude to the many families and friends who are engaged in advocacy for and implementation of truly inclusive play spaces. Creating play spaces for everyone is a sacred work built upon the sacrifices, pain, and sorrow of so many individuals who have experienced life, themselves or with loved ones, void of the freedom to play. Perhaps this book will be another tool for advocacy and education to promote recognition of the need for uninhibited play in our communities. To my remarkable wife, Shinobu, and three fabulous children, I express my deepest love and thanks for the support they have and continue to provide along this journey.

Chad

We would also like to thank Donna Magnani for her guidance and good humor throughout the writing process.

ABBREVIATIONS AND ACRONYMS

AAP   American Academy of Pediatrics
ACE   adverse childhood experience
ADA   Americans with Disabilities Act
ADAAG   Americans with Disabilities Act Accessibility Guidelines
ADHD   attention-deficit/hyperactivity disorder
AOTA   American Occupational Therapy Association
APHA   American Public Health Association
ART   attention restoration theory
ASTM   American Society for Testing and Materials
BMI   body mass index
CPSC   Consumer Product Safety Commission
CPSI   certified playground safety inspector
FBNA   family-based nature activities
ICF   International Classification of Functioning, Disability, and Health
IDEA   Individuals with Disabilities in Education Act
NCA   Norval Community Association
NRPA   National Recreation and Park Association
PIP   pour in place
SRT   stress reduction theory
UN   United Nations
UNISEF   United Nations Children's Fund
WHO   World Health Organization

1

INTRODUCTION

Get Outside!

Long accepted as common knowledge, the concept that being outside benefits the body and mind, is now well supported by an ever-increasing body of research evidence. Studies from a range of design, health care, and education professions validate the health and wellness benefits associated with interacting with nature for both adults and children. These benefits include reduced stress, improved attention and sense of belonging, increased sense of positivity and resilience, reduced obesity, and decreased blood pressure and heart rate, to name just a few (Cordoza et al., 2018; Dean et al., 2018; Diamant & Waterhouse, 2010; Dyment & Bell, 2008; Keniger et al., 2013; Mainella et al., 2011; Roberts et al., 2020).

For children in particular, participation in outdoor activities, including play, is associated with reduced symptoms associated with attention-deficit/hyperactivity disorder (ADHD); an increased sense of restoration, mastery, and resilience; and reduced body mass index (BMI; Berger & Lahad, 2009; Berto et al., 2015; Brown & Summerbell, 2008; Di Carmine & Berto, 2020; Kuo & Faber Taylor, 2004; Wells & Evans, 2003). Positive findings such as these have led the American Public Health Association (APHA, 2013) to advocate that a healthy and active lifestyle is supported by access to nature, and for state and federal agencies to prioritize access to outdoor opportunities.

Sadly, not every child is given equal opportunities to get outside and play, including 8-year-old (let's call her Carina), a little girl with physical challenges with whom Amy worked. Carina loves being around her peers, and when she found out that a group of friends was going to meet at a new playground, she asked her mom to take her there. With some trepidation, Mom agreed, hoping that this time the playground would be at least accessible enough for Carina to join in the play.

DOI: 10.4324/9781003193890-1

Too many times, Carina had been the unintended outcast, sitting on the sidelines in her wheelchair. She was left needing help to ascend a ramp to nowhere-fun or playing with a broken hand spinner on the ground while watching her friends climb to the top of the play structure, slide down, and swing to the sky. Maybe this time it would be different, Mom thought. A new park, a new vision, perhaps? Before even getting Carina out of the van, she looked at the play space and realized that this time would be no better than the other experiences: The playground felt like many others—them and us spaces—with only a small nod to children with disabilities. Nothing felt equal. Instead of subjecting Carina to yet another disappointment, a deflated Mom said to Carina, "Hey, instead of playing, let's go and get some ice cream. It's a perfect day for it." So, they did.

How was that right and just? Despite research and advocacy supporting access to nature, barriers—including the built environment—prevent some children from experiencing all that being outdoors provides. Why does this matter? It matters for all the Carinas of the world. It matters for everyone.

Play

Play is a primary role of childhood. The United Nations (UN) High Commission for Human Rights recognized the vital contribution of play to healthy development and play as the right of every child (UN Office of the High Commissioner, 1990). Outdoor play supports physical, cognitive, sensory, and social-emotional development. Playing in nature provides opportunities for children to move, explore, negotiate, communicate, take risks, be creative and curious, test their physical limitations, and nurture their senses and self-esteem, self-determination, resilience, and assertiveness skills (Furey et al., 2009; Klein et al., 2018; Milteer & Ginsburg, 2012).

All children deserve myriad opportunities to play. The best play happens when the built environment is optimized for all children, regardless of their skill or ability level. Accessibility of public spaces requires compliance with the Americans with Disabilities Act (ADA) Accessibility Guidelines (ADAAG), which set minimum requirements for creating a space, including play spaces usable for persons with disabilities (U.S. Department of Justice, 2010). Despite play being a primary childhood role, children with physical, social-emotional, sensory, or communication challenges run the risk of feeling unwelcome and disconnected when trying to navigate a play space with limited or segregated accessibility (Ripat & Becker, 2012). Caregivers with disabilities also may feel marginalized. Incorporating ADAAG guidelines but going beyond its scope, inclusive play spaces are carefully and thoughtfully planned and designed for everyone. An inclusive design process focuses on usability by holistically integrating easy-to-use, convenient, and safe features that promote participation in play. The most impactful play spaces are those that welcome diversity and are equitable and intuitive.

What You Will Find in This Book

In this book, we share reasons and practical strategies to design outdoor places that embrace inclusivity. We begin by presenting the predominant physiological, social-emotional, language, and cognitive benefits of being in nature—for anyone at any time. The conversation proceeds to explore the fascinating history of outdoor play and types of play, and how both directly affect child development. A developmental milestones chart is included in Chapter 4, "Typical Childhood Development," to help guide age-appropriate design decisions when creating outdoor play spaces for children and youth.

The conversation progresses to a discussion of the importance of the eight sensory systems—touch (tactile), smell (olfactory), see (visual), hear (auditory), taste (gustatory, as appropriate), move (proprioception), balance (vestibular), and internal functioning (interoception)—and how each, working together, can assist with self-regulation, the ability to manage and control one's emotions and behavioral responses (Martini et al., 2016). All these skills are necessary for children to learn and experience. What better places to nurture the sensory systems than in the outdoors, within the context of play? As discussed in detail in Chapter 6, "Inclusive Design," consideration in design guidelines for the eight sensory systems is essential in inclusive play space design because providing a variety of sensory elements enables children to self-regulate and engage in activities most effectively.

With this foundation, we move on to defining inclusion and discuss inclusive play and how it is, at a minimum, a necessary consideration in designing outdoor play spaces to ensure every child, regardless of age, ability, cultural or socioeconomic background, race, or gender, is afforded a fair and equitable opportunity to play. Detailed design guidelines intended for children from birth to 18 years are presented to inspire all who work with and care for and about children to create inclusive play spaces that nurture and enrich all aspects of child development. Relevant case studies are presented in each chapter to illustrate concepts. No matter who is designing inclusive outdoor play spaces, at the core we are all older children—curious about, exploring, and learning from the world. When we tap into our intuitive understanding for great play, we can help make more inclusive outdoor play spaces for others. We hope this book inspires you to do just that.

Inclusive play space design is a thorough and sensitive approach that extends beyond considering the needs of children with visual, auditory, and cognitive disabilities. It looks to meet the needs of a broader spectrum of challenges, including children with invisible disabilities such as those from cognitive, sensory integrative, and mental health. According to the UK Commission for Architecture and the Built Environment, "Inclusive design is about making places everyone can use." As an approach, it "aims to remove the barriers that create undue effort and separation. It enables everyone to participate equally, confidently and independently in everyday activities" (Fletcher, 2006, p. 3). When applied to play spaces, inclusive design is comprehensive and equitable; it fosters resilience and enables every child, caregiver, and family to use these spaces as they want and need to.

References

American Public Health Association. (2013). *Improving health and wellness through access to nature*. https://www.apha.org/policies-and-advocacy/public-health-policy-statements/policy-database/2014/07/08/09/18/improving-health-and-wellness-through-access-to-nature

Berger, R., & Lahad, M. (2009). A safe place: Ways in which nature, play and creativity can help children cope with stress and crisis; establishing the kindergarten as a safe haven where children can develop resiliency. *Early Child Development and Care, 180*, 889–900. https://doi.org/10.1080/03004430802525013

Berto, R., Pasini, M., & Barbiero, G. (2015). How does psychological restoration work in children: An exploratory study. *Journal of Child and Adolescent Behavior, 3*(3), 1–9. https://doi.org/10.4172/2375-4494.1000200

Brown, T., & Summerbell, C. (2008). Systematic review of school-based interventions that focus on changing dietary intake and physical activity levels to prevent childhood obesity: An update to the obesity guidance produced by the National Institute for Health and Clinical Excellence. *Obesity Reviews, 10*(1), 110–141. https://doi.org/10.1111/j.1467-789X.2008.00515.x

Cordoza, M., Ulrich, R. S., Manulik, B. J., Gardiner, S. K., & Fitzpatrick, P. S. (2018). Impact of nurses taking daily work breaks in a hospital garden on burnout. *American Journal of Critical Care, 27*(6), 508–512. https://doi.org/10.4037/ajcc2018131

Dean, J. H., Shanahan, D. F., Bush, R., Gaston, K. J., Lin, B. B., Barber, E., Franco, L., & Fuller, R. A. (2018). Is nature relatedness associated with better mental and physical health? *International Journal of Environmental Research and Public Health, 15*(7), 1–18. https://doi.org/10.3390/ijerph15071371

Diamant, E., & Waterhouse, A. (2010). Gardening and belonging: Reflections on how social and therapeutic horticulture may facilitate health, wellbeing, and inclusion. *British Journal of Occupational Therapy, 73*(2), 84–92. https://doi.org/10.4276/030802210X12658062793924

Di Carmine, F., & Berto, R. (2020). Contact with nature can help ADHD children to cope with their symptoms. The state of the evidence and future directions for research. *Visions for Sustainability, 14*, 1–11. https://doi.org/10.13135/2384-8677/4883

Dyment, J. E., & Bell, A. C. (2008). "Our garden is colour blind, inclusive and warm": Reflections on green school grounds and social inclusion. *International Journal of Inclusive Education, 12*(6), 1–15. https://doi.org/10.1080/13603110600855671

Fletcher, H. (2006). *The principles of inclusive design: They include you.* Commission for Architecture and the Built Environment. https://www.designcouncil.org.uk/fileadmin/uploads/dc/Documents/the-principles-of-inclusive-design.pdf

Furey, M., Tedder, C., Welsh, J., & Wilson, E. (2009, August 31). Promoting accessible playgrounds. *OT Practice, 14*(15). http://www.aota.org/-/media/Corporate/Files/Secure/Publications/OTP/2009/OTP%20Vol%2014%20Issue%2015.pdf

Keniger, L. E., Gaston, K. J., Irvine, K. N., & Fuller, R. A. (2013). What are the benefits of interacting with nature? *International Journal of Environmental Research and Public Health, 10*, 913–935. https://doi.org/10.3390/ijerph10030913

Klein, D., Türk, S., & Roth, R. (2018). Outdoor psychomotor activities: Bringing children to nature. *Advances in Physical Education, 8*(2), 1–7. https://doi.org/10.4236/ape.2018.82022

Kuo, F. E., & Faber Taylor, A. (2004). A potential natural treatment for attention-deficit/hyperactivity disorder: Evidence from a national study. *American Journal of Public Health, 94*, 1580–1586. https://doi.org/10.2105/AJPH.94.9.1580

Mainella, F. P., Agate, J. R., & Clark, B. S. (2011). Outdoor-based play and reconnection to nature: A neglected pathway to positive youth development. *New Directions for Youth Development, 130*, 89–104. https:/doi.org/10.1002/yd.399

Martini, R., Cramm, H., Egan, M., & Sikora, L. (2016). Scoping review of self-regulation: What are occupational therapists talking about? *American Journal of Occupational Therapy, 70*(6), 7006290010p1–7006290010p15. https://doi.org/10.5014/ajot.2016.020362

Milteer, R. M., & Ginsburg, K. R. (2012). The importance of play in promoting healthy child development and maintaining strong parent-child bond: Focus on children in poverty. *Pediatrics, 129*(1), e204–e213. https://doi.org/10.1542/peds.2011-2953

Ripat, J., & Becker, P. (2012). Playground usability: What do playground users say? *Occupational Therapy International, 19*, 144–153. https://doi.org/10.1002/oti.1331

Roberts, A., Hinds, J., & Camic, P. M. (2020). Nature activities and wellbeing in children and young people: A systematic literature review. *Journal of Adventure Education and Outdoor Learning, 20*(4), 298–318. https://doi.org/10.1080/14729679.2019.1660195

United Nations Office of the High Commissioner. (1990). *Convention on the rights of the child.* https://www.ohchr.org/en/professionalinterest/pages/crc.aspx

U.S. Department of Justice. (2010). *2010 ADA standards for accessible design.* http://www.ada.gov/regs2010/2010ADAStandards/2010ADAstandards.htm

Wells, N., & Evans, G. (2003). Nearby nature: A buffer of life stress among rural children. *Environment & Behavior, 35*, 311–330. https:/doi.org/10.1177/0013916503035003001

2

NATURE AND HEALTH

Introduction

We assume that many of you reading this book believe in, enjoy, and/or care about nature. For those who may need convincing, this chapter will provide insight into the relationship between nature and overall health. We represent the "all of the above" category because nature means a lot to our families and us. Recently, Amy's son David was asked to provide an updated bio about himself for a new job. As she read it, Amy was struck by his statement about hobbies, which, except for cooking, all involved nature: hiking, rafting, archery, and running. Nature always has been a part of the family's life, beginning with gardening at their first home and creating that first batch of compost to which David proclaimed, "Look, we remade the earth!" This inherent love for nature in many of us is overwhelmingly supported by research, a small portion of which we here gladly share with you.

Nature and Health; Health and Nature

Terms such as nature interactions, nature contact, nature impact, and nature connection are often used—and just as often used interchangeably—to describe humans' relationships with nature. Take a moment to reread the four terms we just presented. Are they the same? Although all four are similar and equally important in that they link people with nature, they are, in fact, profoundly different. *Nature interaction* and *nature contact* are encounters or actions, such as walking in the woods, lapping around a track in an urban park, weeding the garden, looking out the window at a view of treetops, dipping your toes and fingers in a cool lake, or building sandcastles with family. These encounters and actions may happen nearby, farther away, in a groomed environment, or even in a wild and untamed space. These are good things!

DOI: 10.4324/9781003193890-2

Nature impact is the feeling factor of the experience—the positive or negative effect it has on someone. *Nature connection* is several levels deeper. It is the profound emotional attachment, the "Yes, this is right" bond we feel when we encounter nature that makes us feel good, very good. The impact is strong, positive, and highly preferential; more than likely, we want much more of it. On the surface, weeding the garden is an interaction or contact and can be impactful because it makes a tidier space. However, it can also make us feel happier, calmer, and mentally restored. Physiologically, it can reduce blood pressure and cortisol (a stress hormone) levels. How wonderful—feeling better in mind and body. This connection to nature is so vital that green spaces could be considered a *social determinant of health*. It is a nonmedical health factor that influences and is part of "the conditions in which people are born, grow, live, work, and age" (World Health Organization [WHO], 2021, para. 1).

Understanding the research on how nature improves health and well-being is of foremost importance in designing inclusive outdoor play spaces for children of all ages and abilities. The research can also be the rationale for educating reluctant clients about why these spaces are invaluable. Additionally, the literature on nature and health offers guidance on how thoughtful design can catalyze children to move beyond *nature contact* to *nature connection* and draw them to these spaces time and again. The research we explore provides some of this information.

In this chapter, we look at health and explore the myriad health and wellness benefits for children and adults identified through *contact* and *connection* with nature. Happily, there is already a great deal of research on the topic, with more published regularly. As you read this chapter, think about the *nature contacts* you had today and in the past week and month and whether they became *nature connections*. What was it about these experiences that led to this more profound, more meaningful relationship? Most importantly, how do they make you feel?

Health

The WHO (2006) defined *health* as "a state of complete physical, mental and social well-being and not merely the absence of disease or infirmity" (p. 1). This definition considers the holistic nature of health, acknowledging that health depends on multiple factors within and external to the self. Although not expressly stated in that definition, health can be thought of as a dynamic and fluid process strongly influenced by the many relationships we have with social and physical environments. Considering health in the ways we navigate these environments to function most effectively and engage in life opens the door for creative solutions to solve complex health-related issues (Day et al., 2012). For this book, it is the outdoor environments that can provide support for physical, social-emotional, and cognitive health and well-being.

The international classification of functioning, disability, and health (ICF) is the WHO's (2001) "framework for measuring health and disability at the individual and population levels" (para. 3). The ICF considers the "dynamic products of one's current health state, functioning, lived experiences, and his or her interactions with the sociopolitical [e.g., attitudes, policies, laws] and physical [built and created] environments in which s/he live, work, and participate" (Day et al., 2012, p. 2282). As the WHO (2001) emphasized, the environments we live in can support health—and reduce disability—or they can impede or obstruct it.

People from diverse geographical locations, races, cultures, age and social groups, gender identifications, and ability levels experience discrepant levels of health. These levels may be referred to as inequalities or inequities. A *health inequality* is some health variance across individuals or groups. In contrast, a *health inequity* is a type of inequality representing an unjust disparity in health. Differences that can be measured across or by social groupings (e.g., race, age, ability, or gender) are health inequalities. An example is that younger people tend to enjoy better health than older adults. However, preventable and unjust differences, such as limited access to clean water or vaccinations, are *health inequities* (Arcaya et al., 2015). An example of health inequity that stems from limited resources is varying infant mortality rates among people in different social, economic, racial, or ethnic groups within the same country (Medical News Today, 2021). As we discuss in this chapter, nature influences health for the better. Whether health inequalities and inequities are, at worst, profound or, at best, absent, nature helps to heal.

In sum, health is not a unidimensional construct. Good health depends on myriad social and physical/built environmental experiences we encounter. These experiences provide, limit, or do not provide health equity and equality. The role nature plays in health experiences is indisputable. Let's review why that is the case.

Nature as Health

It is time to go bold. The complex connection between humans and the natural environment is essential to our being and existence (Day et al., 2012; Martin et al., 2020). Provocative? Not at all. In fact, one could say that nature is health, and health is nature. Nature–health connections apply to all social groups—to everyone—throughout life. According to the APHA (2014),

> protecting and restoring access to nature in different spheres of people's lives, among those of all ages, social groups, and abilities, can alleviate some of the most important problems in public health, including obesity, stress, social isolation, injury, and violence.
>
> *(para. 2)*

Research validates these benefits. Anecdotal reports dating to ancient Greek and Roman times and contemporary evidence point to the validity of the essential relationship between nature and health. We start this section with a historical overview of nature and health.

Nature and History

Early humans needed nature for survival and subsistence; it offered sources of shelter, food, water, and clothing (Keniger et al., 2013). Written records dating back to the 2nd century BCE prepared by Roman poets, agronomists, physicians, and politicians noted the important relationship between the body and nature as a key to health (Baker, 2018). Later, when survival no longer depended entirely on nature, private and public green spaces and gardens in Greece, Egypt, and Persia became places to experience well-being and sources of health care (Day et al., 2012). The sensory smells, sights, tastes, textures, and sounds experienced in natural environments were understood to change bodily *humors* (four liquids: blood, yellow bile, black bile, and phlegm) for the better. Later, as population sizes and densities increased, gardens were used as places of respite from busy urban centers (Baker, 2018).

The urbanization of society eventually led to a significantly decreased reliance on nature for subsistence and survival (Keniger et al., 2013). Fortunately, nature—or its modifications—can coexist with an urbanized modern society. Frederick Law Olmstead, the "father" of landscape architecture, designed (for example) New York City's Central Park and the Boston Common as places for the community to glean benefits from natural settings. Interestingly, Olmstead acknowledged the potential for public green spaces to reduce crime, which 21st-century research has shown to, in fact, be the case (Day et al., 2012; Kuo & Sullivan, 2001).

Contemporary lifestyles make regular *contact*, much the less *connection*, with nature challenging, to say the least (Igarashi et al., 2014; Twohig-Bennett & Jones, 2018). Many people living in the industrialized world go about their daily lives disconnected from nature. They spend most of their time inside, not moving nearly as much as needed to prevent ill health (Beyer et al., 2018; Stigsdotter et al., 2010). Increased urbanization, longer workdays, looming expectations to maintain constant interaction on social media, ever-present personal safety concerns, and mounting pressure to succeed have widely supplanted the basic *nature connections* we need for health and well-being.

Developing an Evidence Base

Roger Ulrich conducted the first evidence-based study linking nature and health in the early 1980s. In this seminal study, Ulrich (1984) found that among patients recovering from gall bladder surgical procedures, those with hospital-window views of treetops recovered faster and required less pain medication and nursing staff attention than patients whose views were of a brick wall. Something as seemingly simple as a view of nature accelerated the healing process. A more recent window-view study found that nature views helped minimize the stress and anxiety levels many people experienced during the COVID-19 pandemic (Soga et al., 2020).

Since the publication of Ulrich's (1984) first of many studies, interest in the relationship between nature and physiological and social-emotional health and well-being has expanded exponentially. Shortly, we will explore the current research on nature and health as it applies to adults and children. However, we first examine theories that explain this relationship and apply some nature and health context to the expansive scope of this research.

Several theories and concepts help explain nature and health connections and frame the discussion of nature's relationship to health and well-being. *Biophilia*, humans' hard-wired genetic need and desire to connect with nature (Wilson, 1984), is nurtured through (but not exclusively) childhood experiences, such as being near nature and having caregivers who recognize its value (Broom, 2017). Attention restoration theory (ART), developed by environmental psychologists Rachel and Stephen Kaplan (Kaplan, 1995; Kaplan & Kaplan, 1989), indicates that nature provides restoration from mental fatigue. We experience mental fatigue from engaging in sustained activities, such as hours in front of computer screens or repetitive assembly-job work, and nature allows us to shift from focused attention to involuntary attention. According to ART, this shift refreshes us and replenishes our depleted cognitive capacities. Have you noticed that walking outside in a green environment or gazing out the window at a verdant expanse helped you clear your mind after toiling for hours on a focused task?

A deeper dive into ART reveals four qualities associated with environments that provide attentional restoration. The first, *fascination,* is an environment's capacity to hold your attention. It is important to differentiate between hard and soft fascination. *Hard fascination*, such as with the plethora of neon signs on the Las Vegas Strip, the Ginza in Tokyo, or Times Square in New York City, is not restorative but could be interesting and engaging. On the other hand, *soft fascination*, such as gazing at wispy clouds gliding lazily across the sky or at leaves waving in the wind, is restorative. These nature-related examples draw us in with little or no effort and leave us feeling replenished. The other three features or qualities of ART that provide restoration are *being away* from the pressures of daily life; *extent*, the scope of the environment; and *compatibility*, the match between a person's preferences and the natural environment's features or attributes (Kaplan, 1995; Kaplan & Kaplan, 1989).

Ulrich developed stress reduction theory (SRT; Ulrich, 1984; Ulrich et al., 1991). Unlike ART, which focuses on the cognitive benefits nature can provide, SRT focuses on recovery from stress and improved mood. Interaction with nature, particularly plants, leads to enhanced mood and physiological changes that allow us to relax and "de-stress" (Ulrich, 1984; Ulrich et al., 1991). Contemporary researchers and scholars found that whereas ART and SRT explain the nature–health connection through different lenses, the outcome of both is that nature is health-promoting, a common thread between the two theories.

We introduce the concept of *biophysical ecosystem services* by considering big-picture ways that nature as a construct reduces health risks. *Biophysical ecosystems* are means by which nature changes the physical environment for the better and reduces health risks (Shanahan et al., 2015). One example of this service is plants filtering air pollution and, thus, reducing the rate of respiratory infections.

Another perspective is the green mind theory, which links the mind with the brain and body and connects the body with social and natural environments, such as a walk in the park, that people identify as meaningful. Arguably more interactive than biophysical services, green mind theory has the capacity to positively affect people on the individual and population levels by creating a more sustainable (greener) economy that protects our planet (Pretty et al., 2017). Pretty et al. (2017, p. 12) identified 10 points to activate the green mind theory socially:

- Every child outdoors every day
- Every adult physically active every day
- Every adult learning a new skill or craft throughout life
- Every care home with a garden
- Every hospital redesigned on greener, prosocial principles
- Every natural environment promoted for some human use
- Every person able to access green, social, and talking therapies
- Every person engaged in neighborhood groups for social interaction
- Every kilogram of fossil fuel left in the ground
- Every economy green and prosocial

Of these 10 points, which can you see as applicable to inclusive, outdoor play space design for children and their families? What makes them so?

The APHA (2014) policy statement, "Improving Health and Wellness through Access to Nature," is a testament to why nature must be an essential part of our lives. The paper discusses that almost everyone enjoys increased health and well-being when near nature in the form of "parks, gardens, greenways, naturalized schoolyards and playgrounds, and natural landscaping around homes and workplaces" (para. 3). Table 2.1 provides a snapshot of findings from several health and nature research studies whose results support the APHA policy statement paper, much of which we revisit in greater detail later in this chapter.

One of many significant research findings is that nature experiences can restore emotional and cognitive capacity (Kuo et al., 2019; Scott et al., 2018; Yao et al., 2021). We talk about access to nature being important, but what features of nature elicit health and well-being?

Features such as trees, plants, diverse vegetation, gardens, parks, forests, naturalized play spaces, and water are all understood to contribute to positive health (e.g., APHA, 2014; Toda et al., 2013). Open spaces interspersed with trees are prime opportunities for families to socialize and play with their children. Younger children are drawn to natural spaces as new grounds for exploration, adolescents use natural spaces to spend time with friends, and older adults most enjoy these spaces' opportunities for strolling, viewing, and chatting with friends

TABLE 2.1 Nature and Health Research Findings

Author	Nature and health finding
Mitchell and Popham (2008)	Nature contact reduces overall mortality rate and cardiovascular mortality rate
Mitchell (2013)	Physical activity in natural environments improves psychological health
Lovasi et al. (2008)	Reduced rates of asthma
Hanski et al. (2012)	Reduced rates of allergies
Groenewegen et al. (2012)	Self-reported improvement in health status
Ulrich (1984)	Improved healing occurs when nature is present
Groenewegen et al. (2012)	Increased social connectivity
Tennessen and Cimprich (1995)	Reduced stress
van den Berg and Custers (2011)	
Wells and Evans (2003)	
Cooper (2015)	Improved cognitive skills
Dallimer et al. (2011)	
Han (2009)	
Wells (2000)	
MacKerron and Mourato (2013)	Happiness
Thompson Coon et al. (2011)	Exercising outdoors elicits feelings of happiness, positivity, and reduction in anger and tension
Bell et al. (2008)	Higher levels of nearby green space for children in low-income neighborhoods is associated with lower BMI
Izenstark and Middaugh (2022)	Outdoor play in naturalized areas in childhood is correlated with increased love and appreciation of nature, including environmental stewardship, in adulthood
Ward Thompson et al. (2008)	
Frumkin et al. (2017)	Urban green space provides city dwellers places to relax and destress
Ballew and Omoto (2018)	Improved emotional well-being
Lee et al. (2013)	Improved physiological levels
Neale et al. (2019)	
Roe et al. (2013, 2017)	
Toda et al. (2013)	
Hansen et al. (2017)	Enhanced immune function
Cameron and Hitchmough (2016)	Increased physical activity
Wicks et al. (2022)	

(APHA, 2014). Unlike the sounds, smells, and sights of urban environments, what we experience in green open spaces, including parks, woodlands, and bodies of water, can recharge the body and mind. The most restorative open space environments are nature-rich; although still restorative, the least effective open spaces are athletic playing fields (White et al., 2013).

In terms of health promotion, being in nature encourages physical activity (Araújo et al., 2019; Keskinen et al., 2018). However, the types of nature that inspire people to get out and exercise vary by personal preference. Nature is increasingly recognized as an effective, low-cost therapeutic intervention to improve physical and social-emotional health. These interventions include gardening, exercising in nature, or journaling, to name a few. They are particularly effective for people with long-term chronic conditions, such as diabetes and depression (Howarth et al., 2020), and crucial during the COVID-19 pandemic, when the safest (and often only) means of achieving positive health was outdoor recreation (Javelle et al., 2021; Soga et al., 2020). Using nature as a therapeutic intervention presents an interesting opportunity for designers and planners to create different "sub" environments within a single space to appeal to a wider range of preferences. These sub-environments might include walking trails in densely planted areas, gentle walking routes around a pond, open fields for running, built play spaces, and slow, meandering paths through a sensory garden.

Contact with nature is more than a determinant of health. Importantly, it can—and has been—a relatively inexpensive public health intervention on a population-wide level (Capaldi et al., 2015; Kuo, 2015). A large-scale UK study determined that the health gap between the richest and poorest in the population was smallest when access to green spaces was available nearby (Mitchell & Popham, 2008). Even limited access to green spaces appears to lower a person's risk for fatal diseases; using green spaces to walk and relieve stress may be the common factor in lowering this risk. Subsequently, determining how much time exposure is needed to achieve positive health outcomes for the public remains important for green space planning (Shanahan et al., 2015).

Cognitive Benefits

What is your go-to escape tactic when you feel your brain cannot process one more thing? Did you think immediately of something linked to nature in some way? That is terrific if you did; you are not alone. From a therapeutic perspective, interacting with nature has few or no side effects. For many, it is easily accessible and helps the thought process (Berman et al., 2008). A growing body of evidence is finding that exposure to natural environments also leads to cognitive gains (Schertz & Berman, 2019), and short-duration doses of nature, such as looking at views of nature or brief walks in parks, help redirect attention and improve memory (Kuo et al., 2019). Nature experiences do not require directed attention in what Schertz and Berman (2019) referred to as a *bottom-up approach*. Nature itself draws us in. In contrast, bottom-up urban experiences—screeching brakes, honking horns, blaring music—often require direct attention to keep us safe and alert. These findings align with ART.

For children in particular, nature experiences can positively affect cognition. The literature identified some fascinating findings. Studies from the late 20th and early 21st centuries showed that children perform better on objective cognition measures, such as attention and memory, after exposure to nature and green spaces (Faber Taylor & Kuo, 2009; McCormick, 2017; Wells et al., 2015). We review the takeaways from several of these studies (see Figure 2.1).

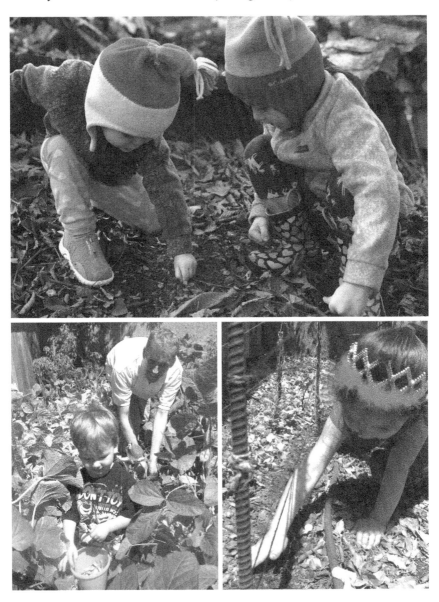

FIGURE 2.1 Curious and engaged in nature-rich exploration. Credit- author and Julie Stevens.

In an experimental study in 2017, children who took a nature walk and then were administered cognitive assessments scored higher on memory and attention tests than children whose walk took them through an urban scape (Schutte et al., 2017). A yearlong study of memory and inattentiveness in 7- to 10-year-old children found a positive association between exposure to green spaces and cognitive skills (Dadvand et al., 2015). Other studies related the density of greenness around children's homes and the green experiences they encounter on their routes to and from school to higher memory and attentional behavior levels (Dadvand et al., 2015; Markevych et al., 2014). Dadvand and colleagues (2015) and Markevych et al. (2014) also linked improved cognition with increased green space exposure duration and lower air pollution levels. The cleanest possible air and more nature on school grounds and everywhere else, truly matter. In short, the greener, the better.

A large national survey studied parents of children diagnosed with ADHD. It found that, regardless of severity level, gender, or socioeconomic status, children who spent at least 20 minutes a day outside in naturalized environments (rather than indoor or outdoor built environments) demonstrated reduced ADHD symptoms, including improved focus and attention (Kuo & Faber Taylor, 2004). Does this harken memories of our mothers telling us, "Just go outside and play?" Comparative to Kuo and Faber Taylor's (2004) seminal study, their ensuing study showed that children with attentional challenges who walked in a park—versus an urban or residential area—showed improved concentration equivalent to the peak effect of extended-release methylphenidate, a medication often prescribed for children with ADHD (Faber Taylor & Kuo, 2009, p. 405). The bottom line appears to be that a dose of nature can be effective medicine.

How does the knowledge that nature enhances children's learning and focus pertain to design? Schools can be designed with greener schoolyards that include plants, trees, shrubs, vegetable gardens, and naturalized and built play spaces. Curricula can be developed to focus on nature in school and the community. Perhaps most importantly, outdoor recess—often eliminated in current curricula—can return as a pivotal part of the day in the life of a young learner.

Participating in school-garden programs can empower children to become more comfortable eating the produce they grow and educating their families on the value of eating fresh fruits and vegetables (McCormick, 2017). One way to improve the quality of an indoor classroom is to green it—by including plants and, if budgets allow, installing green walls. Elementary-school children demonstrated improved cognitive development, including working memory and attentional focus, in classrooms with green walls and greened areas close to the school grounds (Hall & Knuth, 2019; van den Berg et al., 2017). Further, greened classroom features in elementary schools foster a sense of physical comfort, increase attendance, and "improve student's behavior . . . to be enjoyed by teachers and students" alike (van den Berg et al., 2017, p. 806). An important takeaway is that nature is not simply an amenity but a necessity that enhances learning (Schertz & Berman, 2019).

Physical and Physiological Health Benefits

Research about the benefits of nature on physical and physiological health referred to factors such as strength, motion, movement, endurance, heart rate, blood pressure, and nervous system response. As you will read, nature experiences positively influence all these factors for children and adults. The case continues to build for more nature, much more nature, in our daily lives to increase the potential for being and remaining healthy and well.

We begin this section on physical and physiological health with some large-scale thinking. For the most part, we live in an urbanized society. That means we deal daily with many stressors like overstimulation from sights and sounds, large crowds of people, pollution, exhaust fumes, all forms of traffic, and crime (Keniger et al., 2013). These stressors can elicit negative physiological responses, such as increased blood pressure, higher sympathetic (fight-flight-or-freeze) nervous system activity, and even sweaty palms. Nature can buffer the impact of resultant urban overload (Keniger et al., 2013).

It is well known that where we live affects our health. Tree density matters for the express purpose of supporting nature and health connections. People living in neighborhoods with a higher density of trees on their streets indicate higher perceptions of overall health and significantly lower levels of chronic conditions such as stroke, diabetes, high cholesterol, cardiac disease, obesity, and BMI (Dadvand et al., 2014; Hall & Knuth, 2019; Lovasi et al., 2013). Even enhancing a residential home environment with ornamental container plantings led to self-perceptions of reduced stress and increased happiness and pride in the home. These self-reported outcomes were supported by positive physiological changes, such as improved cortisol levels and sleep patterns for at least 3 months after installing the plants (Chalmin-Pui et al., 2021).

Let's overlay a public health population perspective on Chalmin-Pui et al.'s (2021) findings: If ornamental plantings can reduce stress for the residents of homes, then greening on a larger scale—to neighborhoods and municipalities—expands the potential for improved mental health to an even greater extent. Installing edible food gardens in urban areas may be a creative solution to both green up and mitigate health disparities. These gardens provide a source of nutrition and an opportunity to be physically active in nature and introduce contact with commensal bacteria that improve the immune system (Stoltz & Schaffer, 2018). *Commensal microbiota*, often called "good bacteria," live on or in our bodies and help the immune system tolerate, instead of attack, nonthreatening immune events (Rook, 2013; von Hertzen et al., 2011). We increase our exposure to these good bacteria through airborne contact or actual physical contact with soil. Dig on, right?

Physical recovery is another area of interest when discussing physical health. Recovery from serious illnesses or conditions like stroke, multiple sclerosis flare-up, infection, or heart attack can require grueling, tiring physical rehabilitation. This kind of rehabilitation often takes place at inpatient rehabilitation facilities and requires much effort from the patients. Typically, the patients are required to participate in several daily therapy sessions and activities to continue treatment. When therapy is finished for the day or during a break, the patients retreat to their rooms—and rooms with unobstructed window views of nature have long been associated with improved health (Ulrich, 1984).

However, this improvement is contingent, to a degree, upon gender and diagnosis. An interesting research study found that men were more likely than women to experience poorer *mental* health when they stayed in rooms with obstructed window views. When women stayed in rooms with panoramic window views of mountains or a valley, they reported experiencing more ongoing *physical* health than did men with the same views. Linking nature with physical and emotional health, when patients retreat to a room with a nature view, it helps them deal with the emotionally demanding course of physical rehabilitation (Raanaas et al., 2012).

Expanding on the idea that nature is valuable to the rehabilitation process and to being outside, moving therapy outdoors from traditional indoor clinics can positively influence physiological health (Wagenfeld & Marder, 2024). For instance, individuals with fibromyalgia reported feeling less pain and more rested after walking in a mature forest (López-Pousa et al., 2015). People with long-term conditions, such as hypertension, arthritis, emphysema, or diabetes, who participated in gardening activities showed reduced blood glucose, cortisol, heart rate variability, and blood lipid levels (Howarth et al., 2020). In a study of community gardeners, men and women had significantly lower BMI and lower chances of being overweight or obese than their neighbors who were not community gardeners (Hall & Knuth, 2019). Gardening is not only health-promoting and therapeutic but also, for many, a pleasurable and good exercise that improves physical and mental health (Soga et al., 2017). Gardening for at least 1 hour a week improves balance (Chen & Janke, 2012), which is significant for older adults, for whom fall risks are a real concern.

Being outside is therapeutic, and many occupational, physical, recreational, and speech and language therapists use gardening and walking interventions with their patients. Knowing this, designers of outdoor spaces should consider partnering with these therapists to create outdoor therapy clinics. These teams would be a win-win situation for everyone involved—from patients and their families to therapists (Wagenfeld & Atchison, 2014).

Summarily, a multitude of physical and physiological benefits can be experienced through interactions with plants and nature—exercising in, looking at, interacting with, or even simply being near them. A study found that viewing highly aesthetic nature images elicited a more positive affective state than viewing urban images (Meidenbauer et al., 2020). In another study, even short-duration (15-minute) physical activity in nature improved well-being (Han, 2017). Benefits also extend to better quality and length of sleep, a protective factor against chronic illnesses, such as dementia, coronary conditions, asthma, obesity, and diabetes. They increased immune and autonomic nervous system function, decreased the risk of cardiac and respiratory illness, reduced the likelihood of allergies, and improved digestion (Astell-Burt et al., 2013; Brown et al., 2013; Hall & Knuth, 2019; Shanahan et al., 2015; Watson & Moore, 2011; Zhao et al., 2018).

Large-scale studies have associated living close to nature with a reduced risk for long-term health conditions (Amano et al., 2018). Cortisol rates are reduced where there is green space, an important consideration for low-income, marginalized neighborhoods where greenness may be limited or nonexistent (Ward Thompson et al., 2012). Several of these studies showed that reduced stress, an outcome of interacting with nature, increases metabolism rates and insulin secretion and reduces gut inflammation, which reduce the risk and complications of obesity and diabetes (Astell-Burt et al., 2014; Bhasin et al., 2013; Bodicoat et al., 2014). One explanation for these findings is that physical activity in nature is highly preferential, so we want more of it. Logically, the more we exercise, the better health we experience.

Let's circle back to the autonomic nervous system because of its importance in maintaining balance within the body. As mentioned earlier, this system benefits from nature interactions. The *autonomic nervous system* comprises the sympathetic and parasympathetic nervous systems. The *sympathetic nervous system*, often referred to as the fight-flight-or-freeze system, is activated by real or perceived danger, stress, or fear. When engaged, we feel surged with energy; our hearts race, blood pressure increases, and palms sweat; we feel the need to void. Being in a constant fight-flight-or-freeze state degrades the body. It can lead to changes in the immune system, contributing to chronic health conditions (van den Berg et al., 2015). Enter the *parasympathetic nervous system,* sometimes called the rest-and-digest system, whose function is to return the body to a state of homeostasis or balance. Studies found that viewing real nature or images of nature scenes and being in nature, particularly in forest-bathing conditions, activates the parasympathetic nervous system and helps return the body to a more balanced state, including feeling less stressed (Brown et al., 2013; Park et al., 2010). It is increasingly evident that green space experiences trigger positive physiological and endocrine responses (Hall & Knuth, 2019), leading to better health.

Children spend many hours a day inside their homes and, when old enough, inside their schools. Here are a few reasons why both the home and school environments are being looked at as important places where nature belongs. Children with greater access to natural play areas have increased rates of immune-system-supporting bacteria on their skin (Hanski et al., 2012). Contrary to what one might expect, children with asthma who live in homes with a high concentration of vegetation have lower rates of asthma symptoms, asthma attacks, hospital visits, and school absences than children living in public housing that lacks vegetation (Colton et al., 2015). Classrooms without indoor plants are associated with students who experience increased symptoms of ocular discomfort, such as "tired eyes" and nearsightedness, compared to classrooms with plants (He et al., 2015).

School garden programs are increasingly popular for good reasons. For children, they can lead to increased outdoor physical activity; better gut microbiome (microorganisms that live in the intestines) health, which influences immune function; improved mental health, skin conditions, cancer, and autoimmune diseases; lower BMI; and reduced consumption of fast food (Healthline.com, 2021; Skelton et al., 2020; Utter et al., 2016). In other words, when participating in school garden programs, children make better food choices and become healthier. The benefits are even more impressive when school garden programs are part of the educational curriculum.

Green and outdoor play go hand in hand. Physical activity increases when there is access to nearby parks and gardens (Ding et al., 2011; Shanahan et al., 2015). Children tend to engage in more spontaneous physical activity in greener outdoor spaces. Development of gross (large-muscle) motor skills, like running, jumping, balance, and coordination, are enriched through play in nature. One explanation might be that these skills improve when children play outdoors, where there is less predictable terrain than indoors; hence, children must adapt to the varied conditions (Fjørtoft, 2004).

Not all parks are equal, not by a long shot. Investing in parks development or revitalization can lead to environments that appeal to children and give them ample opportunity to be physically active (Hall & Knuth, 2019). The same benefit for children's physical health goes for neighborhood revitalization. For example, a study of 11- to 13-year-olds' activity levels associated higher proportions of trees and green spaces in their neighborhoods with higher rates of physical activity. For each 5% increase in neighborhood greening, there was a 5% increase in the odds that children would be physically active outdoors (Janssen & Rosu, 2015).

As we discuss more in upcoming chapters, today's children do not play outside as often or as long as their caregivers did (Gray et al., 2015). One reason is increased urbanization, which leads to limited opportunities for nature contact. This is worrisome. Living in areas with nearby nature reduces the rates of childhood obesity and time spent in front of screens (Dadvand et al., 2014). Another barrier to outdoor play is caregiver reluctance to allow their children outdoors for safety reasons or because they do not consider it a priority.

This is concerning at every level because, as we have shown, the research is convincing. Being outside is essential for all aspects of health and, equally important, play is a critical part of healthy child development. Playing outside matters. Sedentary behaviors decrease when children are outside. Research found that physical activity is 2.2–3.3 times higher when children play outside (Gray et al., 2015). Being outside gets children moving. However, recess is being eliminated from school curricula in many parts of the world, and formal physical education classes may be held at most once or twice a week. Further, one study found that children sat, on average, 10% more during indoor physical education classes than in outdoor classes (Skala et al., 2012). How is this negative trend contributing to this generation of children's health? It is obviously of the utmost concern.

Social-Emotional Benefits

It is far-reaching and unrealistic to say that every mental health condition can be resolved through connecting with nature. However, it is fair to say that nature exposure promotes health and well-being. Many exciting research studies have and continue to confirm nature's value in improving social-emotional health. Exposure to nature, particularly wetlands, coastal regions, and uplands (high hilly areas), can help restore depleted emotional and cognitive resources (White et al., 2013). In fact, access to high-density green space within a 3-kilometer radius of one's home is a predictor of lower stress levels (van den Berg et al., 2010).

Many research studies confirmed a positive relationship between interactions with nature and social-emotional health benefits for adults. For older adults living in nursing homes, participation in an 8-week indoor-gardening program improved their life satisfaction and sense of social support and connection (Tse, 2010). Although indoor gardening is affirming for older adults, outdoor environments can also benefit them. The moderating effects of environments, specifically attentional and emotional regulation during a run in a park or urban setting, have been studied. The results suggested that runners experienced a heightened sense of restoration following a run in a park versus an urban environment (Bodin & Hartig, 2003; Huang et al., 2022). This is important because it positively correlates the moderating effects of psychological well-being with physical exercise in natural environments.

Nature serves an important purpose for individuals with diagnosed mental health conditions. For instance, inpatients with mental health diagnoses, including major depression, dysthymia, or the depressive phase of bipolar disorder, who participated in a multiweek gardening program showed a persistent reduction in symptoms of depression and rumination and increased attention at a 3-month follow-up (Gonzalez et al., 2010). These findings are especially significant because they show that the impact of nature interventions is lasting—it provides more than a short-term boost. In another study, adults diagnosed with major depressive disorder showed reduced depressive symptoms after walking in nature, even when asked to think about a troubling memory before starting their walk, indicating they did not ruminate (Berman et al., 2012).

There is a relationship between rumination and working memory (Berman et al., 2011). The more we ruminate or fixate on a topic, the less able we are to process information we need now, like memorizing a phone number when we have no pen or paper to write it down, or ready the information for storage in long-term memory. If nature tamps down rumination, that is yet another of its positive attributes.

Social and therapeutic horticulture activities, such as gardening groups, community gardening, or gardening, as therapeutic interventions facilitated by nurses, psychologists, occupational, and recreational therapists can effectively address mental health issues (Sempik et al., 2014). Gardening as a group can promote a sense of belonging and inclusion for marginalized and isolated groups of people (Jakubec et al., 2021; Suh et al., 2021; Truong et al., 2022). These study results are a mere snapshot of the research that continues to be conducted. They validate that, clinically speaking, incorporating nature into therapy regimes benefits social-emotional health. Numerous studies (and, likely, more in process) focused on the general population and showed that even brief nature contact elicited positive emotions and feelings. Repeated contact amplifies that effect (Capaldi et al., 2015). For instance, people who devote more leisure time to nature-related recreational pursuits report a higher level of positivity than those who do not (Young et al., 2021). One example is community gardening because participating in community gardening increases social connectivity, a sense of belonging, and resilience (Okvat & Zautra, 2011; Truong et al., 2022). For many, access to nature by engaging in leisure activities such as community gardening is relatively easy. And it should be: Nature is and must be for all.

As we shared, many people have access to nature in some capacity—their home garden, a nearby park, a reserve, or a community garden. Repeated visits to green spaces are associated with reduced stress; the farther this green space destination is from people's homes, the more stress they experience (Stigsdotter et al., 2010). This is important because self-directed nature interventions, such as walking, sitting, journaling, and meditating outside, are low- to no-cost strategies that improve emotional health and reduce stress (Capaldi et al., 2015).

Let's sit with this for a moment. Without nearby access to green space, much less a preferential one, it is a challenge to get there and reap its benefits regularly. For people who lack this nearby access, it becomes a health disparity that must be addressed because connecting with nature can be a "promising path to flourishing in life" (Capaldi et al., 2015, p. 9) (see Figure 2.2).

Children need to be provided positive experiences with nature early in life to become stewards of the land and to develop love and care for nature as adults (Broom, 2017; Ward Thompson, 2008). Children who enjoy playing outside and in nature and express a love for nature think about nature more positively as adults; children who lack opportunities to play in nature view it more neutrally as adults. This sets a pattern to create an intergenerational disconnection from nature (Broom, 2017; Izenstark & Middaugh, 2022). A nature-neutral caregiver is less likely to encourage and nurture outdoor play with their children than a nature-positive caregiver would be. Generation by generation, nature-neutral children become nature-neutral caregivers. Then, we cannot help but wonder, does nature no longer matter?

Now add this sobering thought: Lacking nature experiences in childhood is risky because high levels of nature exposure during childhood are associated with a lower risk of mental health disorders in adolescence and adulthood. Flipping this, regardless of adjusting for caregiver socioeconomic status, age, history of mental illness, or location, children who grow up with low levels of green space have a

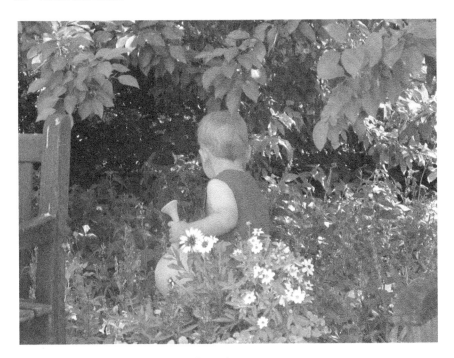

FIGURE 2.2 Nature immersion. Credit- author.

15%–55% higher risk of developing mental illness than their peers who have access (Engermann et al., 2019). What else does the research tell us about nature and social-emotional health?

Often, the strongest connections adults feel with nature reflect their childhood experiences with gardening and other outdoor activities with their families (Izenstark & Ebata, 2019; Izenstark & Middaugh, 2022; Lohr & Pearson-Mims, 2005). In past generations, and with the resurgent interest in home gardening during the COVID-19 pandemic, helping to prepare the garden beds, plant, tend, and harvest has become a central point in family interaction. For the most part, caregivers can provide children opportunities to experience nature through small-scale (e.g., a potted tomato plant) and large-scale (e.g., backyard or allotment) gardening, playing in safe parks, and nature walks. Research showed that consistent nature interaction as part of family time could lead to greater motivation for children to engage in pro-environmental behaviors (Dopko et al., 2019). A longitudinal study showed that having pro-environmental mothers at age 6 years was a positive predictor for children's pro-environmental behaviors at age 18 years (Evans et al., 2018). Children who grow up near nature reap its benefits, including better psychological and social health (Dopko et al., 2019). These experiences matter because childhood exposure to natural outdoor environments may be a protective factor in adulthood (Preuß et al., 2019).

Studies of school-aged children identified valuable benefits that nature offers for social-emotional health. A systematic review of the literature found an overwhelmingly positive relationship between nature interaction and children's behavioral and emotional challenges, particularly for those with ADHD (Vanaken & Danckaerts, 2018). This is an important consideration for educators and school administrators looking to make positive changes in the classroom or learning outside. Installing plants in classrooms was found to be preferential and comforting—not to mention making the room feel more friendly (Han, 2009). Greening schoolyards in low-income urban neighborhoods increased physical activity, enhanced prosocial behaviors, and reduced bullying and gang-related behaviors (Bates et al., 2018). The greater the green space exposure a child has, the greater the reduction in potential emotional and peer-relationship problems (Amoly et al., 2014).

An early and important study of primary-school (Grades 3–5) children found that the amount of nearby nature moderated the impact of stressful life events on the children's psychological well-being and improved their self-worth. The impact of life stress was lowest and self-worth highest among children with the densest levels of nearby nature (Wells & Evans, 2003). That is, nature moderates the impact of stressful life events, such as relocation, being picked on, bullied, or punished in school, and peer pressure, on children's self-worth. Adopting a nature-themed educational curriculum that directly connects children with nature positively affects their self-esteem and sense of well-being (Keniger et al., 2013). The level of greenness on high school campuses directly relates to students' perceptions of restoration: The greener the campus, the more restored the students reported feeling (Akpinar, 2016). Findings are similar for younger children (Bikomeye et al., 2021; Yıldırım & Akamca, 2017).

One of the UN Sustainable Development Goals is to "by 2030, provide universal access to safe, inclusive and accessible, green and public spaces, in particular for women and children, older persons and persons with disabilities" (UN, 2016, para. 2, Goal 11). We hope this will happen—it is imperative. Knowing what we know about nature and health, we must avoid a *biophobia*—a fear of nature—scenario, which can be perpetuated when children lack opportunities to spend positive time in nature (Bixler et al., 1994). Planners, policymakers, and health care professionals on local and national levels must prioritize ensuring that all children have equitable and safe access to green space as a buffer to support sound mental health. What these green spaces look like and ought to contain is an area of study awaiting further research (Engermann et al., 2019). What an opportunity this is—to be a change agent for improving the lives of today's and future generations of children.

Final Thoughts

As we shared in this chapter, from the mid-1980s to date, a surge in research from the design, medicine, public health, and social sciences professions has validated the cognitive, physiological, and social-emotional benefits associated with nature interactions. Nature affects every aspect of ourselves for the better. Active or passive, these experiences have been shown to improve the quality of life for children and adults. They reduce loneliness, stress, and depression and make us more resilient. Being in green spaces helps us think better, focus, concentrate, and even score higher on standardized tests. In nature, our heart rates slow, our blood pressure lowers, and our tendency toward fight-flight-or-freeze reduces. Exercising in nature enhances the effect. So much good comes from nature exposure.

How can we use this research? We can use it to better society. We can work with policymakers and municipal decision-makers to justify and advocate for broad green infrastructure decisions and design and construction with biophilic principles (Hall & Knuth, 2019).

We end this chapter with a final thought about nature's broad and profound influence on human health and well-being. One needs only to reflect on all that nature offers to consider that "nature is vital to us, as it satisfies human physical needs, and aesthetic and spiritual needs" (Broom, 2017, p. 35). We agree wholeheartedly.

BOX 2.1 CASE STUDY: LUCY MAUD MONTGOMERY CHILDREN'S GARDEN OF THE SENSES (FIGURES 2.3–2.5)

Project Information:

Name
Lucy Maud Montgomery Children's Garden of the Senses
Lead Designer
Eileen Foley, Landscape Architect, OALA, CSLA
Location
Norval, Ontario, Canada
Size
3,600 m² or 0.88 acres
Year Built
2016

Description:

The Lucy Maud Montgomery Children's Garden of the Senses is a 0.9-acre immersive garden in Norval, Ontario, Canada. The garden is dedicated to the beloved Canadian author, Lucy Maud Montgomery, who lived in Norval for 9 years. Among other books, she authored the series, *Anne of Green Gables*. In her writings, Montgomery described landscapes and gardens with rich sensory details; hence, this garden pays tribute to her. The Norval Community Association (NCA), a small, volunteer-based, nonprofit organization, which promotes Montgomery's heritage, designed and built the Garden. The Garden is situated within a public park in the town of Halton Hills. The NCA has an agreement with the town for the care of the Garden. The NCA runs hands-on gardening and good related programming for children, older adults, and young adults with intellectual and developmental

Age Group(s)

Children, older adults, and young adults with developmental and intellectual disabilities

disabilities. It also operates an herb garden program in the Garden to promote the health and well-being of its community and help people connect with nature and gain a fuller appreciation of the natural environment through sensory immersive experiences. The Garden is open to the public free of charge.

The sensory gardens are designed to provide diverse nature-rich experiences through their configurations, construction materials, specifically chosen plant material, and other interactive elements that accentuate the senses. A main, level, wayfinding pathway is installed throughout the Garden, and a smaller secondary pathway winds through the sensory gardens. A gazebo beside the Waterfall Garden offers shade and benches for garden programs and art performances. The adjacent Children's Activity Area provides numerous play features: horseshoe reading rocks, a checkerboard log table, a palisade log wall for art, totem poles for painting, hopscotch stepping stones, a log bench for balancing, an accessible sandbox, a children's cottage garden shed, raised planter boxes (Edible Garden), and accessible picnic tables. Other Garden features include fanciful Braille signage, decorative metal benches, and a beautiful bronze statue of a little girl reading a book, presumably one of Lucy Maud Montgomery's!

Website:

- http://gardenofthesenses.com/

Traditional Inclusive Features	Inclusive+ Features

• Accessible path of travel	• Secondary pathway that winds through sensory gardens is paved with concrete, level, and wide.
	• Surfaces within each sensory garden have different degrees of accessibility and tactile walking surfaces to assist with wayfinding for individuals with visual and cognitive impairments.
	  • Keyhole Garden: paving stones
	  • Semicircle Garden: concrete
	  • Sundial Garden: limestone stones
	  • Spiral Garden: screenings

(Continued)

(Continued)

Traditional Inclusive Features	Inclusive⁺ Features
	• Woodland Garden: stepping stones and mulch • Waterfall Garden: mulch and pebble rocks • Edible Garden: screenings • The Garden provides ample opportunities for visitors to choose their own journeys and experience a sense of autonomy and success on their own terms. • Vibrant bright color selections (plants and landscape elements) assist in wayfinding for those with visual and cognitive challenges. • Various seating options, such as raised garden walls for sitting and viewing the gardens, metal benches in the main plaza, benches in the shaded gazebo, and accessible picnic tables, enable visitors to select the one that best meets their needs. • There are varying levels of play opportunities in the Children's Activity Area. • The sandbox is located on a slope, allowing one end of the box to be higher. Wheeled mobility users can roll their wheels under the sandbox and play equitably with standing users. • The raised planter boxes in the Edible Garden are designed for seated gardeners to tend the vegetable and herb plantings. • Multipurpose signage integrates Braille, graphics, and simple text. • The Children's Garden fosters inclusiveness and allows individuals of all ages and abilities to enjoy its treasures.

Remarks:

The garden is widely used for spontaneous activity and multigenerational programming that is loved by children and adults of all ages and abilities. Visitors experience sensory enrichment and the health-promoting benefits of nature on their own terms through an inclusive⁺ journey, exploration, and hands-on interaction with the garden elements. While each of the 10 gardens within the larger garden focus on a particular sensory system, such as the checkerboard garden for sight and the butterfly garden for sound, they all provide other secondarily, nature-rich sensory nurturance. Because the sensory systems guide everything that we do in our lives, these sensory features integrated within the garden enhance the users' experiences multifold.

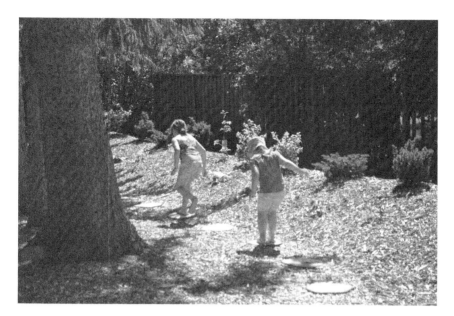

FIGURE 2.3   Girls playing in the Woodland. Credit- Eileen Foley.

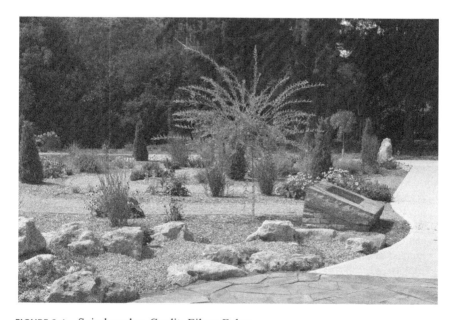

FIGURE 2.4   Spiral garden. Credit- Eileen Foley.

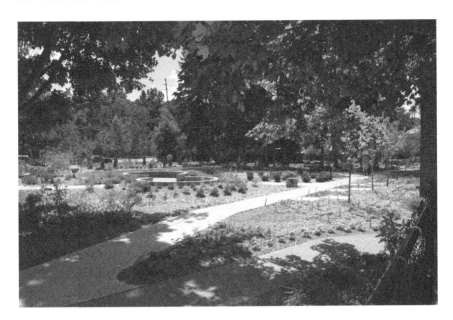

FIGURE 2.5 The main entry. Credit- Eileen Foley.

References

Akpinar, A. (2016). How is high school greenness related to students' restoration and health? *Urban Forestry & Urban Greening, 16*, 1–8. https://doi.org/10.1016/j.ufug

American Public Health Association. (2014). *Improving health and wellness through access to nature.* https://www.apha.org/policies-and-advocacy/public-health-policy-statements/policy-database/2014/07/08/09/18/improving-health-and-wellness-through-access-to-nature

Amoly, E., Dadvand, P., López-Vicente, M., Basagana, V., Julvez, J., Alvarez-Pedrerol, M., Nieuwenhuijsen, M. J., & Sunyer, J. (2014). Green and blue spaces and behavioral development in Barcelona schoolchildren: The BREATHE Project. *Environmental Health Perspectives, 122*(12), 1351–1358. https://doi.org/10.1289/ehp.1408215

Amano, T., Butt, I., & Peh, S.-H. (2018). The importance of green spaces to public health: A multi-continental analysis. *Ecological Applications, 28*(6), 1473–1480. https://doi.org/10.1002/eap.1748

Araújo, D., Brymer, E., Brito, H., Withagen, R., & Davids, K. (2019). The empowering variability of affordances of nature: Why do exercisers feel better after performing the same exercise in natural environments than in indoor environments? *Psychology of Sport and Exercise, 42*, 138–145. https://doi.org/10.1016/j.psychsport.2018.12.020

Arcaya, M. C., Arcaya, A. L., & Subramanian, S. V. (2015). Inequalities in health: Definitions, concepts, and theories. *Global Health Action, 8*(1), Article 27106. https://doi.org/10.3402/gha.v8.27106

Astell-Burt, T., Feng, X., & Kolt, G. S. (2013). Does access to neighborhood green space promote a healthy duration of sleep? Novel findings from 259,319 Australians. *BMJ Open, 3*(8), e003094. https://doi.org/10.1136/bmjopen-2013-003094

Astell-Burt, T., Feng, X., & Kolt, G. S. (2014). Greener neighborhoods, slimmer people? Evidence from 246,920 Australians. *International Journal of Obesity, 38*, 156–159. https://doi.org/10.1038/ijo.2013.64

Baker, P. (2018). Identifying the connection between Roman conceptions of "pure air" and physical and mental health in Pompeian gardens (c. 150 BC–AD 79): A multi-sensory approach to ancient medicine. *World Archaeology, 50*(3), 404–417. https://doi.org/10.10 80/00438243.2018.1487332

Ballew, M. T., & Omoto, A. M. (2018). Absorption: How nature experiences promote awe and other positive emotions. *Ecopsychology, 10*(1), 26–35. https://doi.org/10.1089/ eco.2017.0044

Bates, C. R., Bohnert, A. M., & Gerstein, D. E. (2018). Green schoolyards in low-income urban neighborhoods: Natural spaces for positive youth development outcomes. *Frontiers in Psychology, 9*, Article 805. https://doi.org/10.3389/fpsyg.2018.00805

Bell, J. F., Wilson, J. S., & Liu, G. C. (2008). Neighborhood greenness and 2-year changes in body mass index of children and youth. *American Journal of Preventative Medicine, 35*, 547–553. https://doi.org/10.1016/j.amepre.2008.07.006

Berman, M. G., Jonides, J., & Kaplan, S. (2008). The cognitive benefits of interacting with nature. *Psychological Science, 19*(12), 1207–1212. https://doi.org/10.1111/j.1467-9280.2008.02225.x

Berman, M. G., Kross, E., Krpan, K. M., Askren, M. K., Burson, A., Deldin, P. J., Kaplan, S., Sherdell, L., Gotlib, I. H., & Jonides, J. (2012). Interacting with nature improves cognition and affect for individuals with depression. *Journal of Affective Disorders, 140*(3), 300–305. https://doi.org/10.1016/j.jad.2012.03.012

Berman, M. G., Nee, D., Casement, M., Kim, H., Deldin, P., Kross, E., Gonzalez, R., Demiralp, E., Gotlib, I., Hamilton, P., Joormann, J., Waugh, C., & Jonides, J. (2011). Neural and behavioral effects of interference resolution in depression and rumination. *Cognitive, Affective, & Behavioral Neuroscience, 11*(1), 85–96. https://doi.org/10.3758/s13415-010-0014-x

Beyer, K. M. M., Szabo, A., Hoormann, K., & Stolly, M. (2018). Time spent outdoors, activity levels, and chronic disease among American adults. *Journal of Behavioral Medicine, 41*, 494–503. https://doi.org/10.1007/s10865-018-9911-1

Bhasin, M. K., Dusek, J. A., Chang, B. H., Joseph, M. G., Denninger, J. W., Fricchione, G. L., Benson, H., & Libermann, T. A. (2013). Relaxation response induces temporal transcriptome changes in energy metabolism, insulin secretion and inflammatory pathways. *PloS One, 8*(5), e62817. https://doi.org/10.1371/journal.pone.0062817

Bikomeye, J. C., Balza, J., & Beyer, K. M. (2021). The impact of schoolyard greening on children's physical activity and socioemotional health: A systematic review of experimental studies. *International Journal of Environmental Research and Public Health, 18*(2), 535. https://doi.org/10.3390/ijerph18020535

Bixler, R. D., Carlisle, C. L., Hammitt, W. E., & Floyd, M. F. (1994). Observed fears and discomforts among urban students on field trips to wildland areas. *Journal of Environmental Education, 26*(1), 24–33. https://doi.org/10.1080/00958964.1994.9941430

Bodicoat, D. H., Donovan, G. O., Dalton, A. M., Gray, L. J., Yates, T., Edwardson, C., & Jones, A. P. (2014). The association between neighbourhood greenspace and type 2 diabetes in a large cross-sectional study. *BMJ Open, 4*(12), Article e006076. https://doi.org/10.1136/bmjopen-2014-006076

Bodin, M., & Hartig, T. (2003). Does the outdoor environment matter for psychological restoration gained through running? *Psychology of Sport and Exercise, 4*, 141–153. https://doi.org/10.1016/S1469-0292(01)00038-3

Cooper, A. (2015). Nature and the outdoor learning environment: The forgotten resource in early childhood education. *International Journal of Early Childhood Environmental Education, 3*(1), 85–97.

Broom, C. (2017). Exploring the relations between childhood experiences in nature and young adults' environmental attitudes and behaviours. *Australian Journal of Environmental Education, 33*(1), 34–47. https://doi.org/10.1017/aee.2017.1

Brown, D. K., Barton, J. L., & Gladwell, V. F. (2013). Viewing nature scenes positively affects recovery of autonomic function following acute mental stress. *Environmental Science & Technology, 47*(11), 5562–5569. https://doi.org/ 10.1021/es305019p

Cameron, R. W. F., & Hitchmough, J. (2016). *Environmental horticulture: Science and management of green landscapes.* CABI.

Capaldi, C., Passmore, H.-A., Nisbet, E., Zelenski, J., & Dopko, R. (2015). Flourishing in nature: A review of the benefits of connecting with nature and its application as a wellbeing intervention. *International Journal of Wellbeing, 5*(4), 1–16. https://doi.org/10.5502/ijw.v5i4.449

Chalmin-Pui, L. S., Roe, J., Griffiths, A., Smyth, N., Heaton, T., Clayden, A., & Cameron, R. (2021). "It made me feel brighter in myself": The health and well-being impacts of a residential front garden horticultural intervention. *Landscape and Urban Planning, 205*, Article 103958. https://doi.org/10.1016/j.landurbplan.2020.103958

Chen, T.-Y., & Janke, M. C. (2012). Gardening as a potential activity to reduce falls in older adults. *Journal of Aging and Physical Activity, 20*(1), 15–31. https://doi/org/10.1123/japa.20.1.15

Colton, M. D., Laurent, J. G. C., MacNaughton, P., Kane, J., Bennett-Fripp, M., Spengler, J., & Adamkiewicz, G. (2015). Health benefits of green public housing: Associations with asthma morbidity and building-related symptoms. *American Journal of Public Health, 105*(12), 2482–2489. https://doi.org/ 10.2105/AJPH.2015.302793

Dadvand, P., Nieuwenhuijsena, M., Esnaolaa, M., Fornsa, J., Basagañaa, X., Alvarez-Pedrerola, M., Rivas, I., López-Vicente, M., De Castro Pascual, M., Su, J., Jerrett, M., Querol, X., & Sunyera, J. (2015). Green spaces and cognitive development in primary schoolchildren. *Proceedings of the National Academy of Sciences of the United States of America, 112*(26), 7937–7942. https://doi.org/10.1073/pnas.1503402112

Dadvand, P., Villanueva, C. M., Font-Ribera, L., Martinez, D., Basagaña, X., Belmonte, J., Vrijheid, M., Grazuleviciene, R., Kogevinas, M., & Nieuwenhuijsen, M. J. (2014). Risks and benefits of green spaces for children: A cross-sectional study of associations with sedentary behavior, obesity, asthma, and allergy. *Environmental Health Perspectives, 122*(12), Article 1329. https://doi.org/10.1289/ehp.1308038

Dallimer, M., Tang, Z. Y., Bibby, P. R., Brindley, P., Gaston, K. J., & Davies, Z. G. (2011). Temporal changes in greenspace in a highly urbanized region. *Biology Letters, 7*, 763–766. https://doi.org/10.1098/rsbl.2011.0025

Day, A. M. B., Theurer, J. A., Dykstra, A. D., & Doyle, P. C. (2012). Nature and the natural environment as health facilitators: The need to reconceptualize the ICF environmental factors. *Disability and Rehabilitation, 34*(26), 2281–2290. https://doi.org/10.3109/09638288.2012.683478

Ding, D., Sallis, J. F., Kerr, J., Lee, S., & Rosenberg, D. (2011). Neighborhood environment and physical activity among youth: A review. *American Journal of Preventive Medicine, 41*(4), 442–455. https://doi.org/10.1016/j.amepre.2011.06.036

Dopko, R. L., Capaldi, C. A., & Zelenski, J. M. (2019). The psychological and social benefits of a nature experience for children: A preliminary investigation. *Journal of Environmental Psychology, 63*, 134–138. https://doi.org/10.1016/j.jenvp.2019.05.002

Engermann, K., Bøcker Pedersen, C., Arge, L., Tsirogiannis, C., Mortensen, P. B., & Svenning, J.-C. (2019). Residential green space in childhood is associated with lower risk of psychiatric disorders from adolescence into adulthood. *Proceedings of the National Academy of Science of the United States of America, 116*(11), 5188–5193. https://doi.org/10.1073/pnas.1807504116

Evans, G. W., Otto, S., & Kaiser, F. G. (2018). Childhood origins of young adult environmental behavior. *Psychological Science, 29*, 679–687. https://doi.org/10.1177/0956797617741894

Faber Taylor, A., & Kuo, F. E. (2009). Children with attention deficits concentrate better after walk in the park. *Journal of Attention Disorders, 12*(5), 402–409. https://doi.org/10.1177/1087054708323000

Fjørtoft, I. (2004). Landscape as playscape: The effects of natural environments on children's play and motor development. *Children Youth and Environments, 14*(2), 1–44.

Frumkin, H., Bratman, G. N., Breslow, S. J., Cochran, B., Kahn, P. H., Jr., Lawler, J. J., Levin, P. S., Tandon, P. S., Varanasi, U., Wolf, K. L., & Wood, S. A. (2017). Nature contact and human health: A research agenda. *Environmental Health Perspectives, 125*(7), Article 075001. https://doi.org/10.1289/EHP1663

Gonzalez, M. T., Hartig, T., Patil, G. G., Martinsen, E. W., & Kirkevold, M. (2010). Therapeutic horticulture in clinical depression: A prospective study of active components. *Journal of Advanced Nursing, 66*(9), 2002–2013. https://doi.org/10.1111/j.1365-2648.2010.05383.x

Gray, C., Gibbons, R., Larouche, R., Sandseter, E., Bienenstock, A., Brussoni, M., Chabot, G., Herrington, S., Janssen, I., Pickett, W., Power, M., Stanger, N., Sampson, M., & Tremblay, M. (2015). What is the relationship between outdoor time and physical activity, sedentary behaviour, and physical fitness in children? A systematic review. *International Journal of Environmental Research and Public Health, 12*(6), 6455–6474. https://doi.org/10.3390/ijerph120606455

Groenewegen, P. P., van den Berg, A. E., Maas, J., Verheij, R. A., & de Vries, S. (2012). Is a green residential environment better for health? If so, why? *Annals of the Association of American Geographers, 102*, 996–1003. https://doi.org/10.1080/00045608.2012.674899

Hall, C. R., & Knuth, M. J. (2019). An update of the literature supporting the well-being benefits of plants: Part 2 Physiological health benefits. *Journal of Environmental Horticulture, 37*(2), 63–73. https://doi.org/10.24266/0738-2898-37.2.63

Han, K.-T. (2009). Influence of limitedly visible leafy indoor plants on the psychology, behaviour, and health of students at a junior high school in Taiwan. *Environment and Behavior, 41*(5), 658–692. https://doi.org/10.1177/0013916508314476

Han, K.-T. (2017). The effect of nature and physical activity on emotions and attention while engaging in green exercise. *Urban Forestry & Urban Greening, 24*, 5–13. https://doi.org/10.1016/j.ufug.2017.03.012

Hansen, M. M., Jones, R., & Tocchini, K. (2017). Shinrin-yoku (forest bathing) and nature therapy: A state-of-the-art review. *International Journal of Environmental Research and Public Health, 14*, Article 851. https://doi.org/10.3390/ijerph14080851

Hanski, I., von Hertzen, L., Fyhrquist, N., & Haahtela, T. (2012). Environmental biodiversity: Human microbiota and allergy are interrelated. *Proceedings of the National Academy of Sciences, 109*(21), 8334–8339. https://doi.org/10.1073/pnas.1205624109

He, M., Xiang, F., Zeng, Y., Mai, J., Chen, Q., Zhang, J., & Morgan, I. G. (2015). Effect of time spent outdoors at school on the development of myopia among children in China: A randomized clinical trial. *Journal of the American Medical Association, 314*(11), 1142–1148. https://doi.org/10.1001/jama.2015.10803

Healthline.com. (2021). *The gut microbiome.* https://www.healthline.com/health/gut-health# signs-and-symptoms

Howarth, M., Brettle, A., Hardman, M., & Maden, M. (2020). What is the evidence for the impact of gardens and gardening on health and well-being: A scoping review and evidence-based logic model to guide healthcare strategy decision making on the use of gardening approaches as a social prescription. *BMJ Open, 10*(7), e036923. https://doi.org/10.1136/bmjopen-2020-036923

Huang, D., Jiang, B., & Yuan, L. (2022). Analyzing the effects of nature exposure on perceived satisfaction with running routes: An activity path-based measure approach. *Urban Forestry & Urban Greening, 68,* Article 127480. https://doi.org/10.1016/j.ufug.2022.127480

Igarashi, M., Ikei, H., Song, C., & Miyazaki, Y. (2014). Effects of olfactory stimulation with rose and orange oil on prefrontal cortex activity. *Complementary Therapies in Medicine, 22*(6), 1027–1031. https://doi.org/10.1016/j.ctim.2014.09.003

Izenstark, D., & Ebata, A. T. (2019). Why families go outside: An exploration of mothers' and daughters' family-based nature activities. *Leisure Sciences, 44*(5), 559–577. https://doi.org/10.1080/01490400.2019.1625293

Izenstark, D., & Middaugh, E. (2022). Patterns of family-based nature activities across the early life course and their association with adulthood outdoor participation and preference. *Journal of Leisure Research, 53*(1), 4–26. https://doi.org/10.1080/00222216.2021.1875274

Jakubec, S. L., Szabo, J., Gleeson, J., Currie, G., & Flessati, S. (2021). Planting seeds of community-engaged pedagogy: Community health nursing practice in an intergenerational campus-community gardening program. *Nurse Education in Practice, 51,* Article 102980. https://doi.org/10.1016/j.nepr.2021.102980

Janssen, I., & Rosu, A. (2015). Undeveloped green space and free-time physical activity in 11 to 13-year-old children. *International Journal of Behavioral Nutrition and Physical Activity, 12*(1), 26. https://doi.org/10.1186/s12966-015-0187-3

Javelle, F., Laborde, S., Hosang, T., Metcalfe, A. J., & Zimmer, P. (2021). The importance of nature exposure and physical activity for psychological health and stress perception: Evidence from the lockdown period during the COVID-19 pandemic 2020 in France and Germany. *Frontiers in Psychology, 12,* Article 425. https://doi.org/10.3389/fpsyg.2021.623946

Kaplan, S. (1995). The restorative benefits of nature: Toward an integrative framework. *Journal of Environmental Psychology, 15*(3), 169–182. https://doi.org/10.1016/0272-4944(95)90001-2

Kaplan, R., & Kaplan, S. (1989). *The experience of nature. A psychological perspective.* Cambridge University Press.

Keniger, L. E., Gaston, K. J., Irvine, K. N., & Fuller, R. A. (2013). What are the benefits of interacting with nature? *International Journal of Environmental Research and Public Health, 10,* 913–935. https://doi.org/10.3390/ijerph10030913

Keskinen, K. E., Rantakokko, M., Suomi, K., Rantanen, T., & Portegijs, E. (2018). Nature as a facilitator for physical activity: Defining relationships between the objective and perceived environment and physical activity among community-dwelling older people. *Health & Place, 49,* 111–119. https://doi.org/10.1016/j.healthplace.2017.12.003

Kuo, F. E., & Faber Taylor, A. (2004). A potential natural treatment for attention-deficit/hyperactivity disorder: Evidence from a national study. *American Journal of Public Health, 94,* 1580–1586. https://doi.org/10.2105/ajph.94.9.1580

Kuo, F. E., & Sullivan, W. (2001). Environment and crime in the inner city: Does vegetation reduce crime? *Environment and Behavior, 33*(3), 343–367. https://doi.org/10.1177/0013916501333002

Kuo, M. (2015). How might contact with nature promote human health? Promising mechanisms and a possible central pathway. *Frontiers in Psychology, 6.* https://doi.org/10.3389/fpsyg.2015.01093

Kuo, M., Barnes, M., & Jordan, C. (2019). Do experiences with nature promote learning? Converging evidence of a cause-and-effect relationship. *Frontiers in Psychology, 10,* Article 305. https://doi.org/10.3389/fpsyg.2019.00305

Lee, C., Ory, M. G., Yoon, J., & Forjuo, S. N. (2013). Neighborhood walking among overweight and obese adults: Age variations in barriers and motivators. *Journal of Community Health, 38,* 12–22. https://doi.org/10.1007/s10900-012-9592-6

Lohr, V. I., & Pearson-Mims, C. H. (2005). Children's active and passive interactions with plants influence their attitudes and actions toward trees and gardening as adults. *HortTechnology, 15*(3), 472–476. https://doi.org/10.21273/HORTTECH.15.3.0472

López-Pousa, S., Bassets Pagès, G., Monserrat-Vila, S., de Gracia Blanco, M., Hidalgo Colomé, J., & Garre-Olmo, J. (2015). Sense of well-being in patients with fibromyalgia: Aerobic exercise program in a mature forest; a pilot study. *Evidence-Based Complementary and Alternative Medicine, 2015,* 1–9. https://doi.org/10.1155/2015/614783

Lovasi, G. S., Quinn, J. W., Neckerman, K. M., Perzanowski, M. S., & Rundle, A. (2008). Children living in areas with more street trees have lower prevalence of asthma. *Journal of Epidemiology and Community Health, 62,* 647–649. https://doi.org/10.1136/jech.2007.071894

Lovasi, G. S., Schwartz-Soicher, O., Quinn, J. W., Berger, D. K., Neckerman, K. M., Jaslow, R., & Rundle, A. (2013). Neighborhood safety and green space as predictors of obesity among preschool children from low income families in New York City. *Preventive Medicine, 57*(3), 189–193. https://doi.org/10.1016/j.ypmed.2013.05.012

MacKerron, G., & Mourato, S. (2013). Happiness is greater in natural environments. *Global Environmental Change, 23*(5), 992–1000. https://doi.org/10.1016/j.gloenvcha.2013.03.010

Markevych, I., Teisler, C., Fuertes, E., Romanos, M., Dadvand, P., Nieuwenhuijsen, M., Berdel, D., Koiletzko, S., & Heinrich, J. (2014). Access to urban green spaces and behavioural problems in children. *Environment International, 71,* 29–35. https://doi.org/10.1016/j.envint.2014.06.002

Martin, L., White, M. P., Hunt, A., Richardson, M., Pahl, S., & Burt, J. (2020). Nature contact, nature connectedness and associations with health, wellbeing and pro-environmental behaviours. *Journal of Environmental Psychology, 68,* Article 101389. https://doi.org/10.1016/j.jenvp.2020.101389.

McCormick, R. (2017). Does access to green space impact the mental well-being of children: A systematic review. *Journal of Pediatric Nursing, 37,* 3–7. https://doi.org/10.1016/j.pedn.2017.08.027

Medical News Today. (2021, April 28). *What are social determinants of health?* https://www.medicalnewstoday.com/articles/social-determinants-of-health#education

Meidenbauer, K. L., Stenfors, C. U. D., Bratman, G. N., Gross, J. J., Schertz, K. E., Choe, K. W., & Berman, M. G. (2020). The affective benefits of nature exposure: What's nature got to do with it? *Journal of Environmental Psychology, 72,* Article 101498. https://doi.org/10.1016/j.jenvp.2020.101498

Mitchell, R. (2013). Is physical activity in natural environments better for mental health than physical activity in other environments? *Social Science and Medicine, 91*, 130–134. https://doi.org/10.1016/j.socscimed.2012.04.012

Mitchell, R., & Popham, F. (2008). Effect of exposure to natural environment on health inequalities: An observational population study. *The Lancet, 372*, 1655–1660. https://doi.org/10.1016/S0140-6736(08)61689-X

Neale, C., Aspinall, P., Roe, J., Tilley, S., Mavros, P., Cinderby, S., Coyne, R., Thin, N., & Ward Thompson, C. (2019). The impact of walking in different urban environments on brain activity in older people. *Cities & Health, 4*(1), 94–106. https://doi.org/10.1080/23748834.2019.1619893

Okvat, H. A., & Zautra, A. J. (2011). Community gardening: A parsimonious path to individual, community, and environmental resilience. *American Journal of Community Psychology, 47*(3–4), 374–387. https://doi.org/10.1007/s10464-010-9404-z

Park, B. J., Tsunetsugu, Y., Kasetani, T., Kagawa, T., & Miyazaki, Y. (2010). The physiological effects of Shinrin-yoku (taking in the forest atmosphere or forest bathing): Evidence from field experiments in 24 forests across Japan. *Environmental Health and Preventive Medicine, 15*(1), 18–26. https://doi.org/10.1007/s12199-009-0086-9

Pretty, J., Rogerson, M., & Barton, J. (2017). Green mind theory: How brain–body–behaviour links into natural and social environments for health habits. *International Journal of Environmental Research and Public Health, 14*(7), Article 706. https://doi.org/10.3390/ijerph14070706

Preuß, M., Nieuwenhuijsen, M., Marquez, S., Cirach, M., Dadvand, P., Triguero-Mas, M., Gidlow, C., Grazuleviciene, R., Kruize, H., & Zijlema, W. (2019). Low childhood nature exposure is associated with worse mental health in adulthood. *International Journal of Environmental Research and Public Health, 16*(10), Article 1809. https://doi.org/10.3390/ijerph16101809

Raanaas, R. K., Patil, G. G., & Hartig, T. (2012). Health benefits of a view of nature through the window: A quasi-experimental study of patients in a residential rehabilitation center. *Clinical Rehabilitation, 26*(1), 21–32. https://doi.org/10.1177/0269215511412800

Roe, J. J., Aspinall, P. A., & Ward Thompson, C. (2017). Coping with stress in deprived urban neighborhoods: What is the role of green space according to life stage? *Frontiers in Psychology, 8*, 1–17. https://doi.org/10.3389/fpsyg.2017.01760

Roe, J. J., Ward Thompson, C., Aspinall, P. A., Brewer, M. J., Duff, E. I., Miller, D., Mitchell, R., & Clow, A. (2013). Green space and stress: Evidence from cortisol measures in deprived urban communities. *International Journal of Environmental Research and Public Health, 10*(9), 4086–4103. https://doi.org/10.3390/ijerph10094086

Rook, G. A. (2013). Regulation of the immune system by biodiversity from the natural environment: An ecosystem service essential to health. *Proceedings of the National Academy of Sciences, 110*(46), 18360–18367. https://doi.org/10.1073/pnas.1313731110

Schertz, K. E., & Berman, M. G. (2019). Understanding nature and its cognitive benefits. *Current Directions in Psychological Science, 28*(5), 496–502. https://doi.org/10.1177/0963721419854100

Schutte, A., Turquati, J., & Beattie, H. (2017). Impact of urban nature on executive functioning in early and middle childhood. *Environment and Behavior, 49*(1), 3–30. https://doi.org/10.1177/0013916515603095.

Scott, J. T., Kilmer, R. P., Wang, C., Cook, J. R., & Haber, M. G. (2018). Natural environments near schools: Potential benefits for socio-emotional and behavioral development in early childhood. *American Journal of Community Psychology, 62*(3–4), 419–432. https://doi.org/10.1002/ajcp.12272

Sempik, J., Rickhuss, C., & Beeston, A. (2014). The effects of social and therapeutic horticulture on aspects of social behavior. *British Journal of Occupational Therapy, 77*(6), 313–319. https://doi.org/10.4276/030802214X14018723138110

Shanahan, D. F., Fuller, R. A., Bush, R., Lin, B. B., & Gaston, K. J. (2015). The health benefits of urban nature: How much do we need? *BioScience, 65*(5), 476–485. https://doi.org/10.1093/biosci/biv032

Skala, K. A., Springer, A. E., Sharma, S. V., Hoelscher, D. M., & Kelder, S. H. (2012). Environmental characteristics and student physical activity in PE class: Findings from two large urban areas of Texas. *Journal of Physical Activity and Health, 9*, 481–491. https://doi.org/10.1123/jpah.9.4.481

Skelton, K. R., Lowe, C., Zaltz, D. A., & Benjamin-Neelon, S. E. (2020). Garden-based interventions and early childhood health: An umbrella review. *International Journal of Behavioral Nutrition and Physical Activity, 17*, 1–19. https://doi.org/10.1186/s12966-020-01023-5

Soga, M., Evans, M. J., Tsuchiya, K., & Fukano, Y. (2020). A room with a green view: The importance of nearby nature during the COVID-19 pandemic. *Ecological Applications, 31*(2), Article e2248. https://doi.org/10.1002/eap.2248

Soga, M., Gaston, K. J., & Yamaura, Y. (2017). Gardening is beneficial for health: A meta-analysis. *Preventive Medical Reports, 5*, 92–99. https://doi.org/10.1016/j.pmedr.2016.11.007

Stigsdotter, U. K., Ekholm, O., Schipperijn, J., Toftager, M., Kamper-Jørgensen, F., & Randrup, T. B. (2010). Health promoting outdoor environments: Associations between green space, and health, health-related quality of life and stress based on a Danish national representative survey. *Scandinavian Journal of Public Health, 38*, 411–417. https://doi.org/10.1177/1403494810367468

Stoltz, J., & Schaffer, C. (2018). Salutogenic affordances and sustainability: Multiple benefits with edible forest gardens in urban green spaces. *Frontiers in Psychology, 9,* Article 2344. https://doi.org/10.3389/fpsyg.2018.02344

Suh, J., Auberson, L., & Ede, S. (2021). Connected backyard gardening as a platform for suburban community building in Adelaide, Australia. *Community Development, 53*(1), 21–38. https://doi.org/10.1080/15575330.2021.1936103

Tennessen, C. M., & Cimprich, B. (1995). Views to nature: Effects on attention. *Journal of Environmental Psychology, 15*(1), 77–85. https://doi.org/10.1016/0272-4944(95)90016-0

Thompson Coon, J., Boddy, K., Stein, K., Whear, R., Barton, J., & Depledge, W. H. (2011). Does participating in physical activity in outdoor natural environments have a greater effect on physical and mental wellbeing than physical activity indoors? A systematic review. *Environmental Science & Technology, 45*(5), 1761–1772. https://doi.org/10.1021/es102947t

Toda, M., Den, R., Hasegawa-Ohira, M., & Morimoto, K. (2013). Effects of woodland walking on salivary stress markers cortisol and chromogranin A. *Complementary Therapies in Medicine, 21*(1), 29–34. https://doi.org/10.1016/j.ctim.2012.11.004

Truong, S., Gray, T., & Ward, K. (2022). Enhancing urban nature and place-making in social housing through community gardening. *Urban Forestry & Urban Greening, 72*, Article 127586. https://doi.org/10.1016/j.ufug.2022.127586

Tse, M. M. Y. (2010). Therapeutic effects of an indoor gardening programme for older people living in nursing homes. *Journal of Clinical Nursing, 19*, 949–958. https://doi.org/10.1111/j.1365-2702.2009.02803.x

Twohig-Bennett, C., & Jones, A. (2018). The health benefits of the great outdoors: A systematic review and meta-analysis of greenspace exposure and health outcomes. *Environmental Research, 166*, 628–637. https://doi.org/10.1016/j.envres.2018.06.030

Ulrich, R. S. (1984). View through a window may influence recovery from surgery. *Science, 224*, 420–421. https://doi.org/0.1126/science.6143402

Ulrich, R. S., Simons, R. F., Losito, B. D., Fiorito, E., Miles, M. A., & Zelson, M. (1991). Stress recovery during exposure to natural and urban environments. *Journal of Environmental Psychology, 11*, 201–203. https://doi.org/10.1016/S0272-4944(05)801847

United Nations. (2016). *The sustainable development goals report*. UN DESA. https://unstats.un.org/sdgs/report/2016/the%20sustainable%20development%20goals%20report%202016.pdf

Utter, J., Denny, S., & Dyson, B. (2016). School gardens and adolescent nutrition and BMI: Results from a national, multilevel study. *Preventive Medicine, 83*, 1–4. https://doi.org/10.1016/j.ypmed.2015.11.022

Vanaken, G. J., & Danckaerts, M. (2018). Impact of green space exposure on children's and adolescents' mental health: A systematic review. *International Journal of Environmental Research and Public Health, 15*(2668), 1–17. https://doi.org/doi:10.3390/ijerph15122668

van den Berg, A. E., & Custers, M. H. G. (2011). Gardening promotes neuroendocrine and affective restoration from stress. *Journal of Health Psychology, 16*, 3–11. https://doi.org/10.1177/1359105310365577

van den Berg, A. E., Maas, J., Verheij, R. A., & Groenewegen, P. P. (2010). Green space as a buffer between stressful life events and health. *Social Science & Medicine, 70*(8), 1203–1210. https://doi.org/10.1016/j.socscimed.2010.01.002

van den Berg, A. E., Wesselius, J. E., Maas, J., & Tanja-Dijkstra, K. (2017). Green walls for a restorative classroom environment: A controlled evaluation study. *Environment and Behavior, 49*(7), 791–813. https://doi.org/10.1177/0013916516667976

van den Berg, M., Wendel-Vos, W., van Poppel, M., Kemper, H., van Mechelen, W., & Maas, J. (2015). Health benefits of green spaces in the living environment: A systematic review of epidemiological studies. *Urban Forestry & Urban Greening, 14*, 806–816. https://doi.org/10.1016/j.ufug.2015.07.008

von Hertzen, L., Hanski, I., & T. Haahtela, T. (2011). Natural immunity: Biodiversity loss and inflammatory diseases are two global megatrends that might be related. *EMBO Reports, 12*(11), 1089–1093. https://doi.org/10.1038/embor.2011.195

Wagenfeld, A., & Atchison, B. (2014). "Putting the occupation back in occupational therapy": A survey of occupational therapy practitioners' use of gardening as an intervention. Open Journal of Occupational Therapy, 4(2), Article 4. https://doi.org/10.15453/2168-6408.1128

Wagenfeld, A., & Marder, S. (2024). *Nature-based allied health practice: Creative and evidence-based strategies*. Jessica Kingsley Publishers.

Ward Thompson, C., Aspinall, P., & Montarzino, A. (2008). The childhood factor: Adult visits to green spaces and the significance of childhood experience. *Environment and Behavior, 40*, 111–143. https://doi.org/10.1177/0013916507300119

Ward Thompson, C., Roe, J., Aspinall, P., Mitchell, R., Clow, A., & Miller, D. (2012). More green space is linked to less stress in deprived communities: Evidence from salivary cortisol patterns. *Landscape and Urban Planning, 105*, 221–229. https://doi.org/10.1016/j.landurbplan.2011.12.015

Watson, D. L. B., & Moore, H. J. (2011). Community gardening and obesity. *Perspectives in Public Health, 131*(4), 163–164. https://doi.org/10.1186/1476-069X-8-S1-S6

Wells, N. M. (2000). At home with nature: The effects of nearby nature on children's cognitive functioning. *Environment & Behavior, 32*, 775–795. https://doi.org/10.1177/00139160021972793

Wells, N. M., & Evans, G. W. (2003). Nearby nature, a buffer of life stress among rural children. *Environment and Behavior, 35*(3), 311–330. https://doi.org/10.1177/00139160021972793

Wells, N. M., Myers, B. M., Todd, L. E., Barale, K., Gaolach, B., Ferenz, G., Aitkin, M., Henderson, C. R., Tse, C., Ostile Pattison, K., Taylor, C., Connerly, L., Carson, J. B., Gensemer, A. Z., Franza, N. K., & Falk, E. (2015). The effects of school gardens on children's science knowledge: A randomized controlled trial of low-income elementary schools. *International Journal of Science Education, 37*, 2858–2878. https://doi.org/10.1080/09500693.2015.1112048

White, M. P., Pahl, S., Ashbulby, K., Herbert, S., & Depledge, M. H. (2013). Feelings of restoration from recent nature visits. *Journal of Environmental Psychology, 35*, 40–51. https://doi.org/10.1016/j.jenvp.2013.04.002

Wicks, C., Barton, J., Orbell, S., & Andrews, L. (2022). Psychological benefits of outdoor physical activity in natural versus urban environments: A systematic review and meta-analysis of experimental studies. *Applied Psychology: Health and Well-Being, 14*(3), 1037–1061. https://doi.org/10.1111/aphw.12353

Wilson, E. O. (1984). *Biophilia.* Harvard University Press.

World Health Organization. (2001). *International classification of functioning, disability and health.* http://apps.who.int/iris/bitstream/handle/10665/42407/9241545429.pdf;jsessionid=11787488B71FFDFD88E2FE225FC29A5F?sequence=

World Health Organization. (2006). *Constitution of the World Health Organization: Basic documents* (45th ed., supp.). https://www.who.int/governance/eb/who_constitution_en.pdf

World Health Organization. (2021). *Social determinants of health.* https://www.who.int/health-topics/social-determinants-of-health#tab=tab_1

Yao, W., Zhang, X., & Gong, Q. (2021). The effect of exposure to the natural environment on stress reduction: A meta-analysis. *Urban Forestry & Urban Greening, 57*, Article 126932. https://doi.org/10.1016/j.ufug.2020.126932

Yıldırım, G., & Akamca, G. Ö. (2017). The effect of outdoor learning activities on the development of preschool children. *South African Journal of Education, 37*(2), 1–10. https://doi.org/10.15700/saje.v37n2a1378

Young, J., Maxwell, H., & Peel, N. (2021). Leisure meets health: Important intersections and alternative discourses. *Annals of Leisure Research, 24*(3), 275–282. https://doi.org/10.1080/11745398.2020.1836666

Zhao, C., Noble, J. M., Marder, K., Hartman, J. S., Gu, Y., & Scarmeas, N. (2018). Dietary patterns, physical activity, sleep, and risk for dementia and cognitive decline. *Current Nutrition Reports, 7*(4), 335–345. https://doi.org/10.1007/s13668-018-0247-9

3
HISTORY AND VALUE OF OUTDOOR PLAY

Introduction

As we observe children at play, we are constantly amazed by the natural ease with which they explore, create, and envision the world around them. They turn an old tree house into a spaceship under attack by alien beings or surgically pull apart an acorn to discover its weevils and inner secrets. These adventures happen almost effortlessly, regardless of age, gender, culture, race, or socioeconomic status. It should not be surprising that play has always been and remains integral to all cultures worldwide. Evidence of child play has been found in archeological excavation sites dating back many millennia, unrestricted by geography. Play persists across time and generations because it benefits children. It supports development and learning and is a key to experiential learning through a combination of active engagement with the environment and interactions with others (Lai et al., 2018; Yogman et al., 2018).

An increased interest in designing outdoor spaces to nurture play began in the mid-20th century, and that interest remains strong today. What is play? Is it a simple activity in which children spontaneously engage, or is there a more complex side to this hallmark characteristic of childhood (and beyond)? Why do children play? What is in it for them? Do 21st-century children play outside enough? All these questions warrant discussion. We explore these questions and more in this chapter.

What Is Play?

A quick Google search for "what is play" yielded over 13 *billion* hits. Obviously, with those kinds of numbers, a simple definition is difficult to pin down. One

DOI: 10.4324/9781003193890-3

definition that resonates positively for us is that *play* is a primary job or occupation of childhood, as described by the American Occupational Therapy Association (AOTA, 2020). Another splendid description of play is "an imaginative private reality [that] contains elements of make-believe and is nonliteral" (Yogman et al., 2018, p. 2). The International Play Association (1989) described the phenomenon as

- vital to develop the potential of all children
- communication and expression, combining thought and action; it gives satisfaction and a feeling of achievement
- instinctive, voluntary, and spontaneous
- a means of learning to live and not merely pass the time

Play is an inherent process that helps children feel competent and confident; thus, it should be a staple in their daily routines. In an American Academy of Pediatrics (AAP) paper, the following statement notes the importance of play for children, parents, caregivers, and other adults who love, care for, and need to connect with the children in meaningful ways:

> Play is essential to the social, emotional, cognitive, and physical well-being of children beginning in early childhood. It is a natural tool for children to develop resiliency as they learn to cooperate, overcome challenges, and negotiate with others. Play also allows children to be creative. It provides time for parents to be fully engaged with their children, to bond with their children, and to see the world from the perspective of their child.
>
> *(Milteer & Ginsburg, 2012, p. e204)*

Through play, children learn life skills, like moving their bodies, sharing, imaginative thinking, social skills, and creativity (Wagenfeld et al., 2014). Life lessons, such as safety precautions to take when faced with natural disasters and dangerous situations, can be taught through games. Children learn to take risks, experiment, and test their physical, social, and emotional limits in comfortable ways and on their own terms while playing. Physicians Regina Milteer and Kenneth Ginsburg (2012) supported this concept: "Active play is so central to child development that it should be included in the very definition of childhood" (p. e205). On a more clinical note, play—especially within a nurturing caregiver–child relationship—may indirectly affect brain function. It buffers adversity and reduces the impact of toxic stress to levels that support resilience and coping (Committee on Psychosocial Aspects of Child and Family Health et al., 2012).

The concept of *social play* (not just play) is remarkably important. Russian psychologist Lev Vygotsky (1978) studied infant and child behavior for most of his life. He concluded that play is optimal when the social or built environment enables children to be in a zone of *proximal development*, that important stage of being close to mastering a skill yet still needing help from a more capable other (one who has mastered the skill). When children with and without disabilities or challenges play together, there is a natural tendency for positive role modeling to occur. The role models can be change agents for their peers in the proximal development zone, well situated for extra help (Wilkes-Gillan et al., 2016).

Outdoor play is critically important because it actively supports the development of physical, cognitive, and mental health skills (Nijhof et al., 2018; Yogman et al., 2018). A landmark AAP (2006) Council on Sports Medicine and Fitness and Council on School Health (2006) white paper recommended 30–60 minutes of outdoor play or exercise per day. Although additional and more contemporary research overwhelmingly confirmed the value of outdoor play, research on nearly 8,950 preschool children sadly revealed that almost half did not play or exercise outdoors even once daily (Tandon et al., 2012). This downward trend continues (Lee et al., 2021; Tremblay et al., 2015). We cannot stress enough that all children, regardless of skill or ability, deserve to participate in play. In fact, play is so crucial that the seminal 1959 (revised in 1989) UN Convention on the Rights of the Child documented play as a right of every child (UN, 1989)—to which we wholeheartedly agree.

Play is universal from childhood through adulthood and supported by adults in every society and culture (Yogman et al., 2018). There are many types of play, and the forms they take differ among societies. These variations in type and form are based partly on economic conditions, how societies view childhood and value play, cultural and religious beliefs, gender roles, and relationships with the natural world (Roopnarine, 2011). Almost without fail, natural and unplanned environments have proven to be the richest and most satisfying ways to accomplish play (Lester & Russell, 2010). However, for children with disabilities and their families, these spaces can present barriers (intended and unintended), a topic we cover in great detail in Chapter 6, "Inclusive Design," and Chapter 7, "Design Guidelines."

We have established that children need to play, and that action can happen inside—at houses of worship, stores, and markets—and outside in yards, gardens, empty lots, sidewalks, open streets, schoolyards, parks, play spaces, beaches, and woods. If you think about it, play happens pretty much everywhere. Play contributes to all parts of development: cognitive, physical, sensory, and social-emotional. Still, for many children, play does not happen as frequently as it should. Poverty, caregiver stress, violence, trauma, and other adverse childhood experiences (ACEs) influence the quality and quantity of play. Many cultures have a decreased tolerance for risk, and first-hand-rich connections with nature are being lost due to increased urbanization, overscheduling of children, and pressure for academic excellence—all at the expense of important, spontaneous play.

These factors do not even address the added challenges and barriers that children with disabilities and their families face in trying to play, particularly in outdoor, unregulated environments. When provided with a rich range of opportunities for outdoor play that are intentionally inclusive, regardless of situation or circumstance, children and everyone around them are set up for success at the outset.

History of Play

The 19th century saw a rise in the recognition of the value of play and the introduction of play spaces. Until this point, the prevailing Western attitude, aligned with the concept of original sin, was that children were simply small adults whose mischievous behavior could be explained by being essentially evil or misguided (Tremblay, 2010). As values and views changed, children were no longer cast as rebellious but as playful, and play began to be acknowledged as necessary for healthy development (Chudacoff, 2007). This recasting brought to light two significant questions: How should play happen? How should it look? (see Figure 3.1).

Manuals published in the latter part of the 19th century supported this paradigm shift—that children were not small adults who were simply untoward and rebellious but rather acting like "children." They helped caregivers understand the value of play and strike a balance between structured and unstructured play. This "manualization" of play paralleled the movement to end exploitive child labor practices and fill newly found unstructured time with safe, functional play occupations or activities (Chudacoff, 2007). Then and now, children being children tend to reject structured play in favor of play with little or no set rules imposed on them by adults—contrary to the common contemporary belief that structured lessons and organized team sports can replace unstructured play.

Play Space History

There are several common play space designs: traditional, contemporary, adventure, and nature. *Traditional* play spaces were the historical mainstay of urban design. Popular from the late 19th to the mid-20th centuries, a traditional play space often included heavy metal swings, teeter-totters, slides, jungle gyms, merry-go-rounds, and sandpits/boxes (Mergen, 2003). As a nod to nature, the Playground Equipment Company introduced the jungle gym in 1933 to replicate trees for climbing. These early traditional play spaces were often located in parklike settings with trees, lawns, and benches for adults to sit and watch their children play.

After World War II, play space design shifted to a *contemporary* theme in which plastic began to replace metal, and textures that more closely replicated nature were introduced into the structures. Play equipment took on forms such as castles, rockets, and forts. Often, these forms were available in smaller-scale versions for residential yard installation.

Some manufactured play equipment evolved to provide many types of play experiences for children with and without disabilities. However, the adventure and nature play community see limitations in entire play spaces furnished with manufactured equipment created for specific purposes. In essence, these pieces of equipment direct what children are to do with them. The drawbacks of manufactured play spaces include saturation and boredom with equipment that cannot change and transform into something different at the child's creative whim. That is, in a nod to

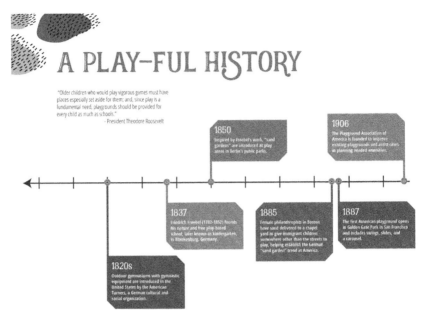

A PLAY–FUL HISTORY

"Older children who would play vigorous games must have places especially set aside for them; and, since play is a fundamental need, playgrounds should be provided for every child as much as schools."
- President Theodore Roosevelt

1850
Inspired by Froebel's work, "sand gardens" are introduced at play areas in Berlin's public parks.

1906
The Playground Association of America is founded to improve existing playgrounds and assist cities in planning needed amenities.

1837
Friedrich Froebel (1782–1852) founds his nature and free play-based school, later known as kindergarten, in Blankenburg, Germany.

1885
Female philanthropists in Boston have sand delivered to a chapel yard to give immigrant children somewhere other than the streets to play, helping establish the German "sand garden" trend in America.

1887
The first American playground opens in Golden Gate Park in San Francisco and includes swings, slides, and a carousel.

1820s
Outdoor gymnasiums with gymnastic equipment are introduced in the United States by the American Turners, a German cultural and social organization.

FIGURE 3.1   A playful history. Credit- Ft. Collins Museum of Discovery.

creativity and risk-taking, children often scale slides and jump off climbing towers, which is not how they were intended to be used. On the other hand, manufactured play equipment is regulated by ASTM International and Consumer Product Safety Commission (CPSC) standards, increasing the likelihood that it is safely usable by a wider range of children than an adventure or nature play space.

The concept of *adventure* play spaces originated in Scandinavia and England as vacant lots furnished with building materials and plants where the children created play worlds, sometimes with adult supervision (Mergen, 2003). Many parts of the world have limited tolerance for adventure play due to its safety and liability concerns. However, there is a "halfway" alternative in nature play spaces.

Nature play spaces replace all or most standard equipment with natural elements like rocks, tree stumps, logs, sand, water, and natural earth forms. Adventure and nature play spaces lend themselves perfectly to loose parts play, which we discuss later in this chapter. There is growing awareness that adventure and nature play spaces offer more opportunities for children to be creative because these spaces lack much structure. Here, children can learn the limits of their bodies more than in traditional or contemporary play spaces. However, these play spaces come with additional perceived risks.

Advocating for Outdoor Play and Play Spaces for Healthy Child Development

The ability to play is important at every phase of development. Play sets the stage to engage in life as an adult; it is the scaffolding or framework for our

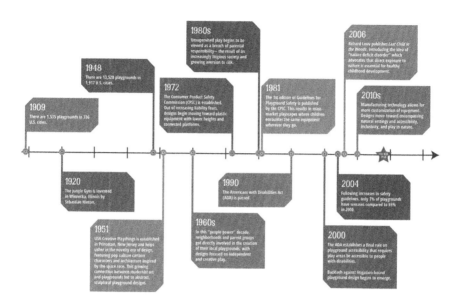

work as adults (Scharer, 2017) because, through play, we gain many life skills. Opportunities to play nurture physical, social-emotional, cognitive, and sensory development. In essence, play helps children thrive (Bento & Dias, 2017), and outdoor play is especially significant for their healthy childhood and adolescent development.

For researchers, outdoor play settings are a natural environment to observe and assess children's developmental skills (Levy & Gottlieb, 1984). As an example, research findings noted that children's and teens' mental health improved after spending time in nature (APHA, 2013; Stone & Faulkner, 2014). For children, the mental health benefits associated with nature engagement include reduced depression and stress and increased resilience, attention, sense of restoration, and overall emotional well-being (Bagot et al., 2015; Barnes et al., 2017; Berger & Lahad, 2010; Faber Taylor & Kuo, 2009; McCormick, 2017; Tillman et al., 2018). Further, social skills can be honed through interactions with natural environments (Miranda et al., 2017). Physical activity levels increase, sedentary behaviors decrease, and, especially for boys, excess weight gain is prevented when children play outdoors (Tillman et al., 2018). Playing in nature provides children with opportunities to move, explore, take risks, test their physical limitations, and nurture their senses (Klein et al., 2018; Wagenfeld et al., 2019). Nature is an ideal environment where children can learn (Acar, 2014). Through play, children engage in trial and error and experience success and failure (Bento & Dias, 2017). Play is, in many ways, the classroom of real life, a place to develop resilience, autonomy, and a keen sense of curiosity.

Participation in outdoor play activities in childhood sets a lifelong course for adulthood engagement with and appreciation for nature. Childhood experiences—home gardening, playing in parks, hiking, and taking nature classes—influence positive environmental stewardship as adults (Hosaka et al., 2018; Lohr & Pearson-Mims, 2005; McFarland et al., 2014). Further, "family-based nature activities (FBNA)" (Izenstark & Ebata, 2016, p. 139)—leisure activities in natural environments, such as hiking and camping—may lead to positive psychological family outcomes. These include a sense of belonging, cohesion, and shared values (Bongaarrdt et al., 2016; Izenstark & Ebata, 2016). Individual benefits associated with FBNA include "reduced stress, positive affect, and increased attentional capacity" (Izenstark & Ebata, 2016, p. 147). In contrast, limited interaction with natural environments in childhood may be associated with poor mental health and decreased interest during adulthood (Preuß et al., 2019).

Despite the family and personal benefits associated with outdoor leisure (Izenstark & Ebata, 2016, 2019; Paggi et al., 2016), factors such as increased screen time (children) and increased urbanization limit engagement with nature-based activities (Heinrichs, 2016). Prioritizing leisure time also can be challenging, and increased screen time and urbanization compound the problem. Children are not getting the recommended 60 minutes of moderate to vigorous outdoor physical activity daily, as the AAP (2006) Council on Sports Medicine and Fitness and Council on School Health (2006) recommend.

The implications for the reduced individual and FBNA time are concerning on multiple levels. On an individual level, outdoor activities are understood to enhance physical and mental health and wellness (Keniger et al., 2013; Sando, 2019) and enrich and nurture families (Izenstark & Ebata, 2016, 2019; Paggi et al., 2016). Despite research showing the benefits of outdoor play, children throughout the world are playing outdoors less than their caregivers did. When they do play, it is often an adult-supervised, structured activity (Stone & Faulkner, 2014).

In response to increased urbanization and the inevitable decline in children's access to nature, the Playground Association of America (now known as the National Recreation and Park Association [NRPA]) was founded in 1906 with a mission to "advance parks, recreation and environmental conservation" (NRPA, n.d.). More than 100 years later, we struggle with the same basic issues: Children are not getting enough time in nature and do not have enough time to play, despite the documented developmental benefits they provide. Mergen (2003) argued that the interplay between nature and play is important for identity formation. If indeed all children deserve the right to play outdoors, then inclusion must be the primary design focus—regardless of the type or theme of the play space, park, or garden—to ensure that all children's needs are addressed.

Stages of Play

Childhood play is divided into six stages beginning at birth. All stages of play are important, and each builds on the one before it. In *unoccupied play*, infants aged 0–3 months learn about their bodies and how it moves. During unoccupied play, a baby makes what appear to be random sensory-motor movements with their arms and legs, like kicking. During *solitary play*, which also begins at birth and lasts until age 2 years, the child is more focused and intentional in activity than during unoccupied play. Solitary play happens because children are not quite ready to play with others. An example is two children playing with their toys, but neither showing interest in the other.

What follows is *spectator* or *onlooker play*. Beginning at about 2½ years, children start watching others play but do not play with them. An example would be a child watching a group of children playing at a water table but from the sidelines. In *parallel play,* which begins at around 3½ years, children play alongside but not *with* each other. An example would be a group of children building their own structures in the sandbox, not working together or sharing their materials. *Associative play* begins at about age 4 years. Although the children may not interact or play together in associative play, they are at least near each other. One example can occur in a climbing structure; some children are climbing, while others are touching, sitting inside, or running around it. By age 4½ years, children begin to engage in *cooperative play*, a stage in which they interact, develop rules, learn the give-and-take of group play, and are interested in the activity. An example might be a game of tag or catch (Parten, 1932).

Types of Play

The academic literature recognizes five types of play: physical play, play with objects, symbolic play, pretend/sociodramatic play, and games with rules (Yogman et al., 2018). We selected six kinds of outdoor play, each of which has application to all five types of play. The outdoor play examples we explore are *risky play, social and dramatic play, intergenerational play, sensory play, loose parts play*, and *nature play*. All play involves some cause and effect, exploration, and cooperation. Here is one outdoor play scenario that illustrates this connection, showing how play may be a compilation of multiple play types:

> *In their wanderings through an empty neighborhood lot, Taylor and Logan come across a large, tall pile of rocks. They cannot pass up the opportunity to scale the pile* (physical play)*, jump off, and then rearrange the rocks and nearby twigs and branches* (play with objects) *into a castle and moat. They must defend it against unwanted visitors* (symbolic play, pretend/sociodramatic play)—*and negotiate who is welcomed into this secret world* (games with rules).

These same types of play scenarios easily apply to other examples of outdoor risky, social and dramatic, intergenerational, sensory, loose parts, and nature play. As you read through the next sections, think about how difficult it is to draw clear lines between what type of play is happening at any moment: Is stringing together a chain of daisies an example of playing with objects or pretend play, planning for it to be a bridge for trolls to cross? Unless we are there to observe, we simply do not know!

Risky Play

After climbing through a weathered window and onto the ledge of a wooden A-frame play structure in the backyard, I (Chad) took a moment to adjust my ingenious (but highly ineffective) grocery bag parachute snuggly against my shoulders. The mere 7-foot drop was no different in my 8-year-old mind and eyes than a 50-foot drop. I was noticeably cautious, and a few encouraging shouts from below were necessary to help build sufficient courage to leap. The plastic grocery bag flapped loudly as the ground approached—much more rapidly than expected! After all, the parachute should have slowed my descent, right? I lived to tell the tale and vividly remember making that leap many more times.

Unbeknownst to me at the time, these, and other types of risks during my youthful playtime were the ultimate training for risk management as an adult. Modern research has revealed that this, along with many other benefits of risky play for all aspects of children's development, is the case in most situations.

What Is Risky Play?

Risky play is universal and observed in all demographics of children. It fills an innate developmental need not met any other way. The crux of risky play is a "child's attempt to manage perceived danger in an environment with the reward of excitement, achievement, and exhilaration" (Kutska, 2013, para. 9).

Benefits of Risky Play

Risk in a play space is essential for children's growth. It creates challenges that provide children opportunities to succeed or fail based on individual reasoning and choices, helping them to learn risk management. *Hazards*, on the other hand, are items or situations that a child is not expected to comprehend, see, or foresee. Risky play has been shown to benefit children's development. It helps them learn to cope with stressful situations, follow through, improve social interaction skills, increase creativity, understand human mortality and their own limitations, recognize areas for improvement, and form positive, proactive attitudes (Brussoni et al., 2015; Gleave, 2008). Other benefits include improved motor skills and cognitive understanding of the environment (Sandseter, 2009a, 2009b) (see Figure 3.2).

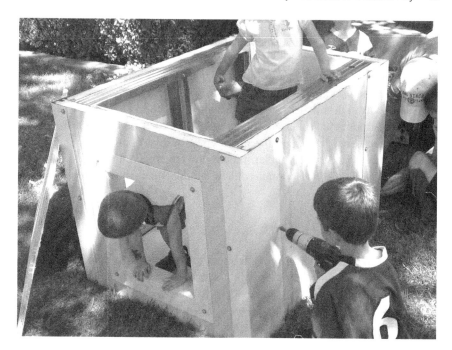

FIGURE 3.2   Risky construction play. Credit- author.

A lack of risk in the play environment could lead to "risk averse" children who never learn to effectively manage everyday situations or children who seek out dangerous locations to experience thrill. Mental health professionals argue that the lack of risk in play can also lead to a lack of resilience and, ultimately, mental health issues resulting in the need for professional intervention (Gleave, 2008). Advocates' arguments for risky play are quite convincing. Some even suggest that risky play is a product of evolution and natural selection, but this has no bearing on why children choose to engage in this form of play every day.

Risky Play from the Child's Perspective

It is common to see risky play in scenarios where the children's skills exceed the opportunities afforded them in play spaces (Sandseter, 2007). This can manifest in a child using equipment in unintended ways, jumping from high places, climbing structures or trees, and mock aggression. One study showed that children's most common and preferred form of risky play was climbing. It did not matter what they climbed—trees, poles, rocks, play climbers, hills, or anything else—as long as the opportunity to climb was there. Second to climbing, children preferred jumping from elevated locations over other forms of play (Sandseter, 2007; Sandseter & Kennair, 2011).

However, the degree to which children are willing to take risks varies greatly. Every child constantly manages their feelings of fear versus anticipated enjoyment and makes a choice. This assessment period ranges from seconds to minutes, depending on the child; some jump right into activities, whereas others hesitate or retreat. Ultimately, children choose to engage in risky play or not based on whether the reward outweighs the risk. It should be noted that children with disabilities are no different from other children in this regard. They benefit as much from risky play and should not be denied the opportunity by overly protective caregivers. Inclusive[+] play spaces, in particular, should provide opportunities for all children to manage risk. Next are descriptions of how children outwardly express their emotions during risky play.

Fear

Much of a child's time during play is spent managing the emotion of fear. This emotion can be recognized primarily by the avoidance or retreat from an activity. Still, other expressions of fear can be observed when a child acts defiantly, freezes in place, becomes defensive or timid, or solicits an adult's help (Sandseter, 2009b). This is a normal, healthy, emotion all children experience at some level and should learn to manage while they are young.

Exhilaration

Exhilaration is the reward the child feels after having accomplished a risky feat they may have been unsure about in the beginning. Children's experiences during risky play border on euphoria; hence, they tend to engage in the same action repetitively to reexperience the original pleasure and excitement (Sandseter, 2009a). This emotion is commonly expressed by laughing, smiling, screaming, yelling, dancing, and engaging in vestibular (rotational/spinning)-oriented play (Sandseter, 2009b).

Borderline Fear

Children often feel out of control or involved in unpredictable situations during play. They tend to be unsure, maybe confused, about the emotions they are feeling. Are they scared, exhilarated, or both (Sandseter, 2009b)? During these times, a child may quickly experience fear followed by exhilaration or vice versa, which is noticeable when the child suddenly stalls or hesitates during play.

Categories of Risky Play

Through interviews and studies of several children's programs in Norway, risky play has been categorized into six main types according to the risk involved (Sandseter & Kennaire, 2011). Not all are found in every play environment.

If they are not, children will instinctively attempt to find ways of experiencing them. A brief list follows:

- Great heights: climbing, jumping, balancing, hanging
- High speed: swinging, sliding, running, biking, skating
- Dangerous tools: cutting, poking, whipping, sawing, lashing, tying
- Dangerous elements: elevation changes, water, fire
- Mock aggression: wrestling, fencing, play fighting
- Disappearing/getting lost: exploring, unknown environments

The research is quite clear on the benefits of risky play and explains it nicely in this statement: "Play is not just about having fun but about taking risks, experimenting, and testing boundaries" (Yogman et al., 2018, p. 2). The task we face as a society now is to determine how to avoid over-sanitizing play environments, minimize regulations, and allow children space to explore and experience while providing safe recreation, free of hazards that could result in serious injury or death. The generations before us understood that accidents happen and are not always bad.

My (Chad's) fearless leaps from rooftops, ledges, and trees (with and without homemade parachutes) did not always end well. I earned my share of bumps, bruises, and even a broken arm. However, these experiences served me well during my early development, as an adult, and eventually as a parent.

Social and Dramatic Play

Although I remember it like it happened yesterday, it has been nearly 30 years since I (Amy) watched my son and his friend Billy engrossed in their social-dramatic play. It was a breezy summer afternoon. The boys were so absorbed in their play that they had no idea I was watching them while I hauled load after load of topsoil to the vegetable garden. They were learning the history of the Indigenous people of the Delaware Valley, where we lived at the time. Intrigued by the Indigenous crafts, food gathering and preserving, and healing practices, the boys were busy transforming our green-bean tepee into a home base for storing the food they had gathered—play food from the sandbox and unripe vegetables harvested from the garden (ouch!).

During a hunt for rabbits to "skin" for their pelts and hang from the tepee "rafters" to preserve for winter, Billy got "hurt" and needed healing. David gently laid Billy on a bed of leaves and opened his imaginary waist pouch. He kneeled over Billy, chanting quiet prayers and waving healing stones from his imaginary pouch over Billy's injured body. Billy was successfully healed, and the play resumed. They shifted to a canoe trip—in a huge box hauled from the garage—along the Delaware River, searching for fish to smoke and reeds to weave into baskets. Hours passed, and the play became increasingly complex with ongoing negotiations about who was doing what. When Billy's dad picked him up, the boys shed an abundance of tears—neither boy wanted to end this magical afternoon's adventure. That was social and dramatic play at its core.

What Is Social Play?

Research tells us that social-emotional functioning has important public health implications throughout the life span. It affects academic performance, mental health, tendency toward criminal behavior, substance abuse, and, as adults, work (Denham et al., 2009, p. i37; Yule et al., 2019). Although it may seem weighty, important life skills learned through social play include reciprocity, group interaction, team play, listening and responding to others' needs and ideas, and conflict resolution (Bauminger-Zviely et al., 2020) (see Figure 3.3).

Children who develop strong social-emotional skills tend to be more adaptive and resilient (Crooks et al., 2020; Denham et al., 2009). Unstructured, child-directed play can help support social skills development (Wilkes-Gillan et al., 2016). Social play is process- rather than product-focused, meaning it does not have an end goal except to be an end unto itself. It need not conform to preconceived

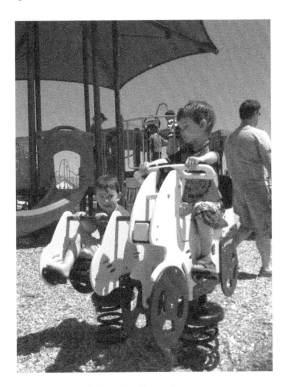

FIGURE 3.3   Spontaneous social play. Credit- author.

rules; it unfolds as the play happens, changing and adapting as the situation and players warrant (Bauminger-Zviely et al., 2020). In social play, children create make-believe scenarios that enable them to take on and practice different roles and perspectives. This kind of play promotes in-the-moment experimenting with themselves, their playgroup, adults, and their environment; thus, they learn social skills in real-time experiential settings (Perren et al., 2019). As they lose themselves in social play, children can better understand their own and others' emotions. They can cope with scary scenarios or roles by inventing and becoming fantasy heroes, which helps them work through issues while playing with peers or adults (Milteer & Ginsburg, 2012).

What Is Dramatic Play?

Dramatic play is social, creative, and complex. It is a world of make-believe that can captivate children for hours. They enter a magical place that allows them to transform themselves and their environment into something novel to suit their needs. Dramatic play behaviors include changing the meaning of things to meet the needs of the moment, taking on the role of someone else to fit the situation, using complex themes motivated by actions and events, and engaging in rich social dialogue to enhance the play event (Robertson et al., 2020, p. 376).

Let's unpack each of these behaviors. *Changing the meaning of things* involves on-the-fly shifting of thought to make objects at hand suit the needs of the play situation. *Taking on the role of someone else* is becoming, in this imaginary play situation, perhaps a revered and admired hero or animal. On the surface, dramatic play may appear simple; in reality, it is a complex world the players negotiate through a series of determined action plans. Dramatic play involves communicating, which, to be inclusive, does not necessarily have to be spoken words. It could be gestures or whatever system the children devise.

Because dramatic play requires communication with others, it involves social interaction and lasts for more than fleeting moments. It can include role-playing—the children acting out what they have seen their parents, caregivers, or other adults do. Dramatic play is social, but alone play also can be dramatic. Likely, we have all observed children engage in solitary play that is quite dramatic and creative. Through dramatic play, children engage deeply with their environment and tackle an insatiable internal drive to master what is real to them. Like any type of play, dramatic play is not a single-benefit experience. Although its primary purpose is to learn and develop social skills, it also involves movement and sensation.

The thinking that comes from social collaboration with peers or adults is different than in alone play (Gupta, 2009). Dramatic play is enriched when an adult or more capable (experienced or older) peer facilitates the process—if they are flexible, attuned to dramatic play scenarios, and step back to allow the children to carry on when or where they are ready. This gentle adult guidance is known as *scaffolding*. The metaphoric space in which the child needs that extra help to master any skill is the *zone of proximal development* (Vygotsky, 1978). Think of the zone of proximal development as "a little help never hurts," an important place if intervening is needed. When done with dignity and respect, scaffolding is an invaluable learning tool.

Dramatic play is a rich and beneficial part of healthy child development. Nevertheless, there is notable concern that today's children do not engage in as much creative, imaginative, and dramatic play as past generations (Goldstein, 2018), coupled with limited outdoor time. This problem is ripe for solutions.

Benefits of Social-Dramatic Play

Vygotsky (1978) recognized dramatic pretend play as crucial—the most influential for learning and overall development. This resounding endorsement is because participating in dramatic play is an ideal way for children to learn and build social skills (Hostettler Scharer, 2017). Whereas all play is important for healthy development, dramatic play has a particularly significant role for self-regulation (Germeroth et al., 2019; Ogan, 2008, as cited in Khomais et al., 2019), an important predictor of academic performance. Self-regulation includes attention, working memory, and inhibitory self-control. Dramatic play helps children develop a *theory of mind*, the awareness that others think differently than they do (Weisberg, 2015). For children, realizing they do not necessarily share the same feelings about a situation as a friend, sibling, or adult is a breakthrough developmental milestone. If dramatic play helps children become more academically and socially competent and proficient, why are we not giving them enough time to play?

Social-Dramatic Play from the Child's Perspective

Dramatic play helps children understand and explain the world they occupy and a safe environment to learn and practice social skills. In dramatic play, children take on new roles and become, for that time, someone or something other than themselves. They use objects symbolically, improvising to suit their needs and support their play (Gao & Hall, 2019). This means using whatever objects or materials are available and engaging in spontaneous dialog to help them learn about who they are and explain the world around them (Brown, 2017, as cited in Gao & Hall, 2019). Here is a great example:

Recently, Amy watched a wonderful dramatic play scenario unfold on a nearby play space. Several school-age children were racing around. Suddenly, one departed the chase line, scrambled up the slide, and beat on the metal with loud bangs that echoed through the small play space. Then came a call to order from the self-appointed leader—resonant bang, bang, bangs. "All of you space creatures, you hear the sound of the 'Gong of Grok.' Now you must gather around and await new orders from me, the King of all Groks."

Dramatic play provides a scaffolding for children to learn from and support each other and creates a world bound only by their imaginations. We invite you to think more about what outdoor dramatic play looks like through the eyes of a child. Here is one more example:

> *It is finally the long-awaited recess time. Five wiggly and restless third-graders rush to the play space and up the ramp to the very tip-top of the play structure. Along the journey, the drama begins. Warp speed travel to the top of the structure—the mission awaits: Protect Earth from an attack of the Hungry Marshmallows, strange creatures from a galaxy far away, whose intention is to rain sugar all over the planet. The children plot the next steps—collect the sugar and transform it into the dreamiest-ever confections. They dance about and make up songs. The drama becomes more complex when the salt-and-pepper people join the play. Suddenly, just as things get exciting, recess ends—but not the story. During recesses for the next week, a rotating cast replays the tale in different ways, and chatter about this strange conundrum abounds in the classroom. Recognizing the value of this dramatic play, the astute teacher infuses the theme into writing, science, and art projects and even facilitates a related cooking activity for the children to enjoy.*

Let's get natural now. Do you recall a time when you and some pals sat astride a log? What came of it? Did you negotiate whether the log was a boat waiting at the dock to be loaded with cargo and then sailed to a faraway land? What was this mysterious cargo? Was it objects you found nearby, like coins (round pebbles)? Did leaves become slices of bread, and sticks become sausages to eat on the journey? Did you help load the cargo? Where were you going on this journey, and how rough was the sea? Were waves crashing into your boat and soaking your clothes? Perhaps you set sail on a day when the sea was glassy and calm with only the tiniest breeze. How did you decide who would row the boat and who would steer? What was the story? How did you decide the rules of the play? When there was conflict, how did you resolve it?

Maybe the boat transformed into a rickety bridge, and crossing it meant a unicorn waited on the other side for you to ride. Who helped you cross the bridge without falling into the "water?" Was it an older peer, a teacher, caregiver, or other adult? Did you race across or crawl on all fours? How did it feel to reach the other side? Do you remember getting there unscathed (or maybe only a bit roughed up)? Continuing the dramatic play, was the unicorn ready to take you to the moon? Did this play last for hours and hours? What memories do you have of transforming a seemingly mundane object into something far more exciting to serve your needs at that moment? Dramatic play involves a great deal of symbolism—and children do know that a rock is not a coin, and a log is not a boat. Nonetheless, their play is a beautiful thing to witness and experience. This is dramatic play.

Intergenerational Play

As a father of young children (Chad), spending afternoons at local parks and play spaces was not uncommon. Several years ago, while chasing my children up, down, and around chutes and ladders, I suddenly noticed a concerning trend that has since fascinated me. Many, if not all, of the other parents, caregivers, and grandparents sat on the sidelines, engrossed in their smartphones and other electronic devices. For all intents and purposes, the play space had become a babysitter, responsible for entertaining the children while the adults performed more "worthwhile" tasks. I was taken aback, perhaps mostly by the fact that I had been guilty of checking emails and updates while "watching" the children play. Why, in so many cases, do only the children recreate in play spaces?

My unscrutinized hypothesis is that adults in our modern play spaces are less engaged because of the lack of intergenerational activities, actual or perceived physical barriers, or a lack of appealing recreational opportunities. Possible solutions to this phenomenon might include creating intergenerational play spaces.

What Is Intergenerational Play?

Intergenerational play is more than a structured formal gathering with people of multiple generations. As Siyahhan et al. (2010) described, "Productive intergenerational play, collaborative work between parent [grandparent] and child . . . is characterized by exchange of expertise between the parent and the child around shared intentions" (p. 429). A truly intergenerational play environment would include diversity in play, complete with interaction and a playful atmosphere. It should involve listening, storytelling, games, and play (Agate et al., 2018). Several common themes occur during intergenerational play, including a desire for adults to share family history with the younger generation; participation in activities that generate a sense of magic, science, and fun; and a generational connection through the use of food (Agate et al., 2018; Davis et al., 2008).

Benefits of Intergenerational Play

The primary intent of intergenerational play is to strengthen the family relationship and respect for and interest in people of different ages. Study after study has shown that such strengthening is most effective through family leisure events that are "unique, shared, interactive, purposive, challenging and requiring sacrifice" (Palmer et al., 2007, p. 446). These opportunities facilitate learning and teaching life skills and lessons, family narratives, and values. Other benefits of intergenerational play are well documented for children and their adult counterparts.

Intergenerational play can dispel myths and preconceptions children feel toward their elders and vice versa. It can help older adults experience a sense of empowerment in their role as "guide" and for children to learn to develop patience and, in some situations, pace themselves with their elders, to be energizing and inspiring, to establish mutual respect and empathy, and to forge emotional connections (Brasileiro et al., 2019). When intergenerational play occurs outside, its benefits include time for shared contemplation and appreciating views, plants, and animals. It is a time for older adults to share stories from their past and for children to find places of connection and common ground with their elders (Harris, 2016). In addition, the health care profession has for some time used intergenerational programming, resulting in benefits such as positive mood changes; improved cognitive, social, and emotional development; and increased levels of engagement for everyone involved, even frail older adults (Listokin, 2011).

Elements of Intergenerational Play

The fundamental elements of intergenerational play revolve around a diverse and flexible palette of activities that appeal to a broad demographic. This does not imply a shotgun approach, cramming as many recreational features as possible into a space. Thoughtful design would create spaces and features that function in versatile ways to engage multiple generations together in an activity. Activities and recreational features should (Spence & Radunovich, 2008)

- provide for a range of ability levels (children, adults, and older adults)
- be easily understandable with instructions or directions
- allow unstructured, creative play guided (not prescribed) by the users
- not create physical, mental, or social barriers like segregated activities or excessive elevation changes
- encourage activities that initiate intergenerational interactions, such as storytelling, playing board games, reading, preparing food, conversing, gardening, and observing

Research related to intergenerational play is lacking; unfortunately, not enough space can be dedicated here to address this topic adequately. That said, the following suggestions based on available research can help guide the implementation of intergenerational play spaces:

- Locate them near community centers, senior centers, teen centers, and schools or in a central location where people of all ages will congregate.
- Use socially and physically inclusive design principles as they apply to people of all ages and abilities, not just to persons with disabilities. This will facilitate intergenerational integration of the activities that occur in the play space.
- Community (vegetable/herb/flower) gardens are a great place for generations to play side by side and learn from each other.
- Include durable outdoor table games, such as checkers, chess, and ping-pong.
- Shade, shade, shade! Provide shade at resting points, in some active areas, and in picnic areas.
- Provide quiet, secluded areas specifically designed for drawing, storytelling, reading jointly, telling jokes, having fun discussions, and observing.
- Include a space for movies and events in the play space.
- Provide accommodations for food. *Grandparents love to buy snacks for their grandchildren!* This includes barbecuing facilities, concessions, and mobile vendors like food trucks and carts.

Intergenerational play is geared toward improved interactions between generations, particularly within the family (Davis et al., 2008). Although important to plan for overall, engaging in or completing *specific* activities is peripheral and should be loosely structured. Play spaces should enrich the quality of social-dramatic play and support positive intergenerational interactions. Outdoor spaces that are safe and enclosed reduce the need for constant site surveillance, so adults can better focus on *playing* with the children. Signage that cues adults on ways to use the play space to enrich the quality of the social interaction can help them step out of the role of parent/grandparent/caregiver/educator and into the role of play partner (Gibson et al., 2020). It moves play into the present moment.

Sensory Play

One of my (Amy) most cherished childhood memories is the summer night my parents decided it was too hot inside and that, despite being long past our bedtimes, we all needed to go outside. Clad in pajamas, the four of us children raced for the door. None of us needed convincing; we all knew something special was about to happen. The air was still, stars twinkled in the sky, and fireflies blinked and fluttered. We did the same, twirling and flying and swooping around the front yard. We listened to the rising and falling sounds of the cicadas. And then, best of all, my dad turned on the sprinkler. We took turns running through it, sitting on it, laying on it, slurping the water, playing the "piano" on the sprinkler's bar, laughing and delighting in this amazing and unexpected sensory treat.

What Is Sensory Play?

Play is inherently a sensory experience. Think about it: Sensory play involves the sensory systems, of which we have eight. Yes, eight: *tactile* (touch), *olfactory* (smell), *gustatory* (taste), *auditory* (hearing), *visual* (seeing), *vestibular* (balance), *proprioceptive* (body position in space and movement), and *interoceptive* (internal regulation). In Chapter 5, "Sensory Integration: Why It Matters," we explore in detail each system and its essential contribution to our daily life functioning. For now, consider the bigger picture of what sensory play is. Maybe a better approach is to consider what sensory play is *not* because, no matter the type of play, some or all sensory systems are involved in some capacity, depending on the child's sensory preferences (Watts et al., 2014). Sensory play can be hands or feet or, more accurately, whole-body play.

On the one hand, sensory activities are well suited for solitary play. Digging, scooping, and pouring soggy sand out of a bucket can be enjoyed alone or in a co-operative social fashion. Children can divide the tasks and work together to build a massive structure and then squish it and start again. When sensory play opportunities exist, either purposely organized by adults or through the imagination and creativity of children who take full advantage of all their play space offers, there is also the opportunity for group learning and problem-solving (Yang & Jia-Wang, 2017).

Benefits of Sensory Play

When playing outside, it is virtually impossible not to smell or touch or—depending on limitations a child may have or the environment imposes—see, hear, taste, and move. In fact, sensory play's scope is so expansive and fluid that it ensures the same experience is never repeated exactly as before (Maynard et al., 2009). Playing outdoors offers many opportunities for children to nourish their sensory systems in ways that best suit their needs and tolerances. Some children will be more eager to be "all in," and others more tentative. We will return to this in Chapter 5, "Sensory Integration: Why It Matters," because knowing more about how our sensory systems affect the way we participate in life is essential when designing inclusive outdoor play spaces.

Loose Parts Play

A while back, while visiting a friend, I (Amy) watched her young daughter, Nelia, build a fairy house from loose parts she had gathered: shells and smooth rocks from the beach; pine needles from the trail to a nearby park; and leaves, seeds, sticks, pinecones, and the like from her yard. Nelia wanted to build a flat house to avoid tripping over it. Considering how to put the pieces of her house together, she cleverly decided to "spear" a leaf in place with the end of a stick and call it a wall. She anchored the sticks in place with pebbles to make them more secure and graced her tree-bark doorway with a curved stick archway. A sweet little flower was one of Nelia's favorite parts of the house; it was special, one of a kind, a treasure found beneath the azalea bush in full bloom—the "only pink part of the house."

Nelia decided her house should be like the one she lives in—with beds and a kitchen so there would be yummy food that she loves for the fairies and sprites to eat. She made a cozy bed of pine needles and created little vessels to store and cook her "food." The vessels, Nelia's "plates and dishes," were small shells filled with grass and water that reminded her of "noodles and sauce" and "dirt like parmesan cheese." Nelia's house was built in an open space, a so-called "vacant" lot, so future fairy-house neighborhoods might soon grace their family garden. After the fairy house was built and enjoyed for a few days, Nelia returned the shells and rocks to the beach and composted everything else.

What Is Loose Parts Play?

Simon Nicholson (1971), an architect and artist, introduced the concept of loose parts in his article "How NOT to Cheat Children: The Theory of Loose Parts" about 50 years ago. Regardless of its identification as a play typology, we can safely assume that loose parts play is one of many ways children have *always* played. Nicholson defined *loose parts* as natural, handmade, or manufactured materials that children can manipulate, experiment with, create, invent, and generally do with whatever they want. Loose parts play comes without set direction; it is limited only by safety, existing environmental constraints, and the far reaches of children's imaginations (Neill, 2013) (see Figure 3.4).

Benefits of Loose Parts Play

Loose parts play is sensory and creative; it works well in solitary, dramatic, and social play. Loose parts play, and opportunities to engage in it, support children's cognitive and social-emotional development (van Dijk-Wesselius et al., 2018). Aside from safety and developmental concerns, the sky is the limit for what children can do and discover with sticks, branches, acorns, mud, leaves, pebbles, bits of string, buckets, strainers, and the like. Although further research is needed to tell us the exact benefits of loose parts play for overall development, we know that it is fun and appears to enhance active and unstructured play (Houser et al., 2016).

Nature Play

The vacant, fallow lot across from my (Chad) home when I was growing up seemed, at my age, to have been there—and neglected—for ages. It was lazily fenced off, so, naturally, it was a main attraction for the neighborhood children. After gaining access to the field of chest-high weeds, we spent hours working in teams to harvest and bundle the weeds to build fortifications and fend off the other children setting up only a dozen feet away. When the forts were sufficiently built in our minds, we

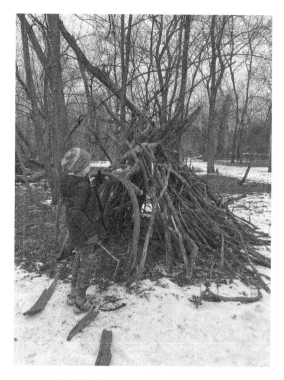

FIGURE 3.4   Loose parts play. Credit- Ryan Durkin.

pulled more weeds out of the ground—at their base to ensure we got the root balls, dirt still clinging—to stock our artillery. We hurled these makeshift dirt-clod missiles between straw bunkers in attempts to overcome the other team's fortifications. I am unsure how long the dusty explosions and laughter-riddled battles persisted, but I remember being filthy, tired, and blissful after each play episode.

What Is Nature Play?

Quite simply, nature play involves engaging in creative activities outside in an environment that has, at a minimum, some nature—ideally, on the wild side. Nature play could be digging a hole to get to the other side of the world, building forts, launching twig boats along a stream, or stealthily slithering like a snake through a patch of tall grass.

Nature's Intrinsic Play Value

First and foremost, nature is constantly changing, providing children with renewable supplies of play materials, sensory experiences, and creeping critters. Play areas integrated with natural elements differ each time a child visits, affording them new experiences. Logically, this type of play area retains its novelty over time and encourages visits more frequently and for longer durations.

Moore et al. (2009) showed that play settings with diverse options could meet the needs of children at all development stages and varying learning styles, personality types, friendship patterns, and cultures. If nature at a play space contains inherent opportunities to learn, experiment, experience, be inspired by, and, in turn, pass this on to other children, it supports Vygotsky's concept of the *zone of proximal development*—that a little bit of help never hurts (Laaksoharju et al., 2012; Vygotsky, 1978). Research also showed that the symbolism children find in nature correlates directly with creative play (Johnson, 2000). Further, it provides an educational experience by promoting hands-on learning and exploration that often do not exist in traditional play spaces. Exploration is a fundamental form of play that provides an innate draw to natural settings, which is essential in helping children understand the surrounding landscape. Natural features, such as inert materials, landforms, seed pods, flowers, grasses, trees, insects, and other wildlife, are curious specimens worthy of childlike exploration and investigation.

Final Thoughts

If we were to sum everything in this chapter into one phrase, it would be that children need to play as though their lives depended on it. Although that might seem an overly dramatic, flashy statement, stop and think about it: Play begins at birth; albeit disorganized, it is nonetheless play. Through play, children learn about themselves, their place in the world, and the world beyond them. They learn to share, make and break rules, and experience risk. In childhood, play is about *learning*. Not every child has opportunities to play. Some are marginalized based on gender, race, ethnicity, socioeconomic status, or physical or mental health challenges and ability, and some by the environment in which they live. Although the impact of not playing enough is bad for all children, those marginalized feel the negative effects more. We end this chapter by sharing this thought:

> All children have the right to safe places to play regularly, during which they develop cognitive, communication, problem-solving, negotiation, and leadership skills. They have the right to engage in safe and regular physical activity that will decrease the incidence of lifelong health disparities. The physically and emotionally healthy children of today will become the productive citizens who will contribute positively to society in the future.
>
> *(Milteer & Ginsburg, 2012, p. e210)*

Hopefully, our collective goal as human beings is to ensure that every child, regardless of who they are or what skills they have, is afforded the right to play often, safely, and well. One inclusive play space at a time, we can change the trajectory and elevate play to where it needs to be in every child's life—front, center, equitable, and available.

BOX 3.1   CASE STUDY: JAKE'S FIELD OF DREAMS (FIGURES 3.5–3.7)

Project Information:

Name
Jake's Field of Dreams
Designer
Unlimited Play, Little Tykes Commercial
Location
Wentzville, MO
Size
1,620 m² or 0.4 acre
Year Built
2018
Age Group(s)
2–5 years, 5–12 years

Description:

Jake's Field of Dreams is an Unlimited Play play space installed at Heartland Park in Wentzville, Missouri. The play space honors the life of Jake Vollmer, who, like many other little boys, dreamed of growing up playing sports. He wanted all children to be able to experience the thrill of playing sports—something he had not had when he passed away in 2012 at the age of 19. The play space includes features such as a double obstacle course for social and gross-motor skill development, a zipline modified with seating to provide postural support, a horizontal bench roller that provides a fun multisensory experience, slides for thrilling movement, a rotating disc climber that offers movement and balance challenges, an at-grade spinner for easy access to rotational movement, interactive dramatic and fine-motor skill panels, a jungle-gym climber for physical and dramatic play, a rocker that provides side-to-side motion, a disc swing for social and sensory play, and a sports sound-reaction game for interactive play.

Websites:

- https://unlimitedplay.org/playground/jakes-field-of-dreams/
- https://www.facebook.com/JakesFieldofDreams/

Traditional Inclusive Features	Inclusive⁺ Features
<ul><li>Accessible path of travel</li><li>Accessible structures</li><li>Accessible swings</li><li>PIP rubber surfacing</li><li>Accessible slides</li><li>Accessible climbers</li></ul>	<ul><li>Bucket-seat zipline with safety harness that accommodates children with limited postural control to sit independently</li><li>Dramatic play sports-based theme conveyed through multisensory features</li><li>Horizontal roller bench that facilitates easy transfer from an ambulatory device such as a wheelchair</li><li>At-grade spinner to experience vestibular motion</li><li>Fine-motor-skill-oriented sports panels to interact with from seated or standing</li><li>Interactive sports-sound game to enrich cause-and-effect play</li></ul>

(Continued)

(Continued)

Traditional Inclusive Features	Inclusive⁺ Features
• Completely fenced perimeter for safety	• Safety zone surface indicators for ease of understanding • Integrated companion seating benches for comfort and socialization • Designed with and built as a unified community • Shade structures to help with temperature and internal regulation

Remarks:

This inclusive community play space is welcoming for children and adults with or without disabilities. The entire $850,000 project was funded exclusively through donations. This project creates an inviting sense of place so families can connect with its unique and recognizable landmark features, making navigation of the space comfortable and organizing. The space is completely fenced, creating a safe environment to reduce the risk of elopement while supporting a primary goal of self-empowerment. This play area has a broadened focus: It does not just contain a typical play structure; it also includes a wide variety of activities to participate in, from slides and spinners to swings and ziplines—and most do not require exit from an ambulatory device. Importantly, the play area's highest elevation is accessible to anyone who wishes to go there. The diversity in play options just mentioned ideally requires a larger developed space. However, the quality of the inclusive⁺ play experience achieved through the Jake's Field of Dreams facility design is much higher because children have the option to choose which activity they would like to participate in and have the opportunity to learn and graduate from one difficulty level to another, eventually experiencing all elements of the play area on their terms.

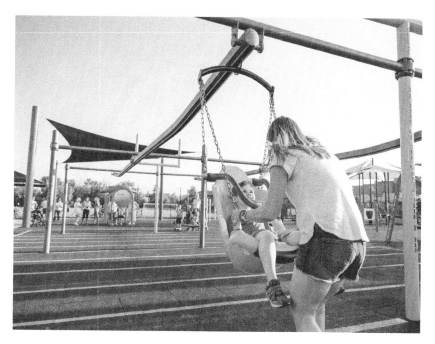

FIGURE 3.5   Affect attunement in play. Credit- Play Power.

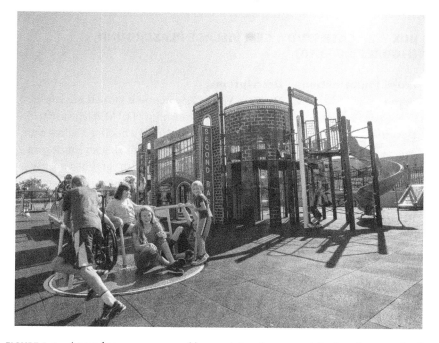

FIGURE 3.6   At grade merry-go-round is a social and sensory rich play element. Credit-
Play Power.

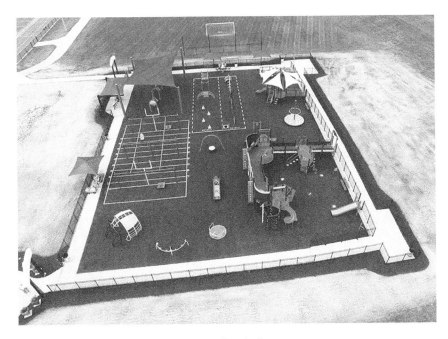

FIGURE 3.7 Bird's eye view. Credit- Natalie Mackay.

BOX 3.2 CASE STUDY: GEM VILLAGE PLAYGROUND (FIGURES 3.8–3.10)

Project Information:

Name
Gem Village Playground
Designer
eMI, O'Dell Engineering, Play Space Creative, Amy Wagenfeld | Design
Location
Kakiri, Wakiso, Uganda
Size
2,020 m² or 0.5 acre
Year Built
2023
Age Group
Birth to 18 years

Description:
The Gem Village Playground is located near the living quarters on the campus of GEM Village in Kakiri, Wakiso, Uganda, a residential school for children with physical and developmental disabilities (most common are cerebral palsy, autism, and/or epilepsy). The play space is explicitly designed to remove the barriers the children faced when attempting to play outdoors. This play area design responds to their disabilities while maintaining the philosophy that the diversity in disabilities should be reflected in the diversity of activities and opportunities for play the built environment affords. The design was created collaboratively between an interdisciplinary team of landscape architects, certified playground safety inspectors (CPSIs), and an occupational therapist from eMI, O'Dell Engineering, Play Space Creative, and Amy Wagenfeld | Design.

Website:

* https://thegemfoundation.com/GemVillage

Traditional Inclusive Features	Inclusive+ Features
• Accessible path of travel • Accommodates children in wheelchairs and children with visual challenges	• Eight sensory-system enrichment features with a range of calming and alerting activities • Artificial turf with sand subgrade to ease physical access and impact attenuation for falls • Low-slope ramps (<5%) reduce the required physical effort to navigate the play area for the children or their nannies to push children in wheelchairs who are unable to propel themselves • The water-play area and all raised-play elements exceed accessibility standards, allowing children to either stand or safely experience all play opportunities without needing to get out of a wheelchair • Universally designed paved sensory trail with simple instructional icons embossed onto the trail to encourage movement, whether seated or on foot • Staff have clear and unobstructed surveillance of the entire play space • Simple and perceptible learning and interactive features • Inclusively accessible and interactive planting features • Nature-based theme to enhance exploratory play options • Multiple cozy spaces for self-regulation and restoration • Integrated grade changes that provide movement challenges • Overarching play approach focused on social connections between the children • Integrated and natural shade options to help with temperature and internal regulation • Adapted interactive art features for cause-and-effect play • Repurposed Boda-Boda motorcycles for culturally relevant adaptive dramatic play

Remarks:

This inclusive[+] play space represents how big ideas can be achieved with a small budget. Using recycled objects and a team of committed volunteers and community organizers, Gem Village Playground is a bright example of how an inclusive[+] play space can come to fruition in even the most extraordinary of circumstances. The emphasis of this design is not on helping the child with a disability adjust to and accept the play environment, but designing the play environment to accommodate the needs, abilities, and strengths of the child. This play environment encourages independence, equality of play opportunity, full participation in play, choice, socialization, and creativity. Everything about the play space is intentional and focused on the needs of the children of GEM Village, including the selected activities, the slopes of the walks, the locations of play elements, and the inclusive[+] design features. This design takes inclusive play to a new level with the addition of a manipulative wall, a sheltered sensory nook, and adapted interactive art. An adaptive sensory walk (focused on self-regulation of sensory input) is another highlight of this project that makes this play space unique among all other play areas in Uganda.

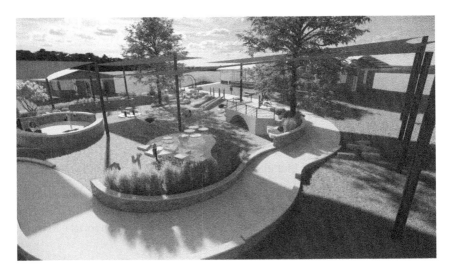

FIGURE 3.8   Bird's eye view of the Upper Terrace. Credit- O'Dell Engineering.

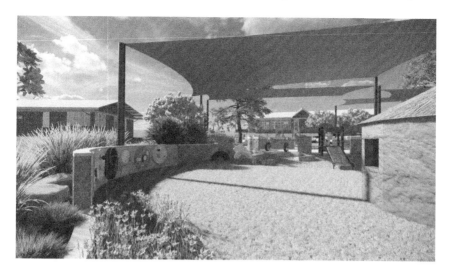

FIGURE 3.9 Lower terrace entry. Credit- O'Dell Engineering.

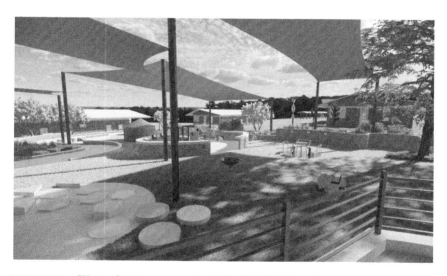

FIGURE 3.10 Water play terrace overlook. Credit- O'Dell Engineering.

References

Acar, H. (2014). Learning environments for children in outdoor spaces. *Procedia: Social and Behavioral Science, 141*, 846–853. https://doi.org/10.1016/j.sbspro.2014.05.147

Agate, J., Taylor Agate, S., Liechty, T., & Cochran, L. J. (2018). "Roots and wings": An exploration of intergenerational play. *Journal of Intergenerational Relationships, 16*(4), 395–421. https://doi.org/10.1080/15350770.2018.1489331

American Academy of Pediatrics. (2006). Active healthy living: Prevention of childhood obesity through increased physical activity. *Pediatrics, 117*(5), 1834–1842. https://doi.org/10.1542/peds.2006-0472

American Occupational Therapy Association. (2020). Occupational therapy practice framework: Domain and process (4th ed.). *American Journal of Occupational Therapy, 74*(Suppl_2), 7412410010–7412410010p87. https://doi.org/10.5014/ajot.2020.74S2001

American Public Health Association. (2013). *Improving health and wellness through access to nature* (Policy No. 20137). https://www.apha.org/policies-and-advocacy/public-health-policy-statements/policy-database/2014/07/08/09/18/improving-health-and-wellness-through-access-to-nature

Bagot, K. L., Allen, F. C. L., & Toukhsati, S. (2015). Perceived restorativeness of children's school playground environments: Nature, playground features and play period experiences. *Journal of Environmental Psychology, 41*, 1–9. https://doi.org/10.1016/j.jenvp.2014.11.005

Barnes, G., Wilkes-Gillan, S., Bundy, A., & Cordier, R. (2017). The social play, social skills and parent-child relationships of children with ADHD 12 months following a RCT of a play-based intervention. *Australian Occupational Therapy Journal, 64*(6), 457–465. https://doi.org/10.1111/1440-1630.12417

Bauminger-Zviely, N., Eytan, D., Hoshmand, S., & Rajwan Ben–Shlomo, O. (2020). Preschool Peer Social Intervention (PPSI) to enhance social play, interaction, and conversation: Study outcomes. *Journal of Autism and Developmental Disorders, 50*(3), 844–863. https://doi.org/10.1007/s10803-019-04316-2

Bento, G., & Dias, G. (2017). The importance of outdoor play for young children's healthy development. *Porto Biomedical Journal, 2*(5), 157–160. https://doi.org/10.1016/j.pbj.2017.03.003

Berger, R., & Lahad, M. (2009). A safe place: Ways in which nature, play and creativity can help children cope with stress and crisis; establishing the kindergarten as a safe haven where children can develop resiliency. *Early Child Development and Care, 180*(7), 889–900. https://doi.org/10.1080/03004430802525013

Bongaarrdt, R., Røseth, I., & Baklien, B. (2016). Hiking leisure: Generating a different existence within everyday life. *SAGE Open, 6*(4), 1–10. https://doi.org/10.1177/2158244016681395

Brasileiro, M. L. S., Moreira, M. A. S. P., de Barros, K. C., & de Medeiros, R. A. (2019). Intergenerational programs among children, young and elderly people with educational emphasis: An integrative review. *HSOA Journal of Gerontology & Geriatric Medicine, 5*, 25–32. https://doi.org/10.24966/GGM-8662/100025

Brussoni, M., Gibbons, R., Gray, C., Ishikawa, T., Sandseter, E. B. H., Bienenstock, A., Chabot, G., Fuselli, P., Herrington, S., Jassen, I., Pickett, W., Power, M., Stanger, N., Sampson, M., & Tremblay, M. S. (2015). What is the relationship between risky outdoor play and health in children? A systematic review. *International Journal of Environmental Research and Public Health, 12*(6), 6423–6454. https://doi.org/10.3390/ijerph120606423

Chudacoff, H. (2007). *Children at play: An American history*. NYU Press.

Committee on Psychosocial Aspects of Child and Family Health, Committee on Early Childhood, Adoption, and Dependent Care, & Section on Developmental and Behavioral Pediatrics. (2012). Early childhood adversity, toxic stress, and the role of the pediatrician: Translating developmental science into lifelong health. *Pediatrics, 129*(1), e224–e231. https://doi.org/10.1542/peds.2011-2662

Council on Sports Medicine and Fitness and Council on School Health. (2006). Active healthy living: Prevention of childhood obesity through increased physical activity. *Pediatrics, 117*(5), 1834–1842. https://doi.org/10.1542/peds.2006-0472

Crooks, C. V., Bax, K., Delaney, A., Kim, H., & Shokoohi, M. (2020). Impact of MindUP among young children: Improvements in behavioral problems, adaptive skills, and executive functioning. *Mindfulness, 11*(10), 2433–2444. https://doi.org/10.1007/s12671-020-01460-0

Davis, H., Vetere, F., Francis, P., Gibbs, M., & Howard, S. (2008). "I wish we could get together": Exploring intergenerational play across a distance via a "magic box." *Journal of Intergenerational Relationships, 6*(2), 191–210. https://doi.org/10.1080/15350770801955321

Denham, S. A., Wyatt, T. M., Bassett, H. H., Echeverria, D., & Knox, S. S. (2009). Assessing social-emotional development in children from a longitudinal perspective. *Journal of Epidemiology & Community Health, 63*(Suppl_1), i37–i52. https://doi.org/10.1136/jech.2007.070797

Faber Taylor, A. F., & Kuo, F. E. (2009). Children with attention deficits concentrate better after walk in the park. *Journal of Attention Disorders, 12*(5), 402–409. https://doi.org/10.1177/1087054708323000

Gao, Q., & Hall, A. H. (2019). Supporting preschool children's learning through dramatic play. *Teaching Artist Journal, 17*(3–4), 103–105. https://doi.org/10.1080/15411796.2019.1680236

Germeroth, C., Bodrova, E., Day-Hess, C., Barker, J., Sarama, J., Clements, D. H., & Layzer, C. (2019). Play it high, play it low: Examining the reliability and validity of a new observation tool to measure children's make-believe play. *American Journal of Play, 11*(2), 183–221.

Gibson, J. L., Fink, E., Torres, P. E., Browne, W. V., & Mareva, S. (2020). Making sense of social pretense: The effect of the dyad, sex, and language ability in a large observational study of children's behaviors in a social pretend play context. *Social Development, 29*(2), 526–543. https://doi.org/10.1111/sode.12420

Gleave, J. (2008). *Risk and play: A literature review*. Playday. https://www.stichtingoase.nl/literatuur/doc/doc_73.pdf

Goldstein, T. R. (2018). Developing a dramatic pretend play game intervention. *American Journal of Play, 10*(3), 290–308.

Gupta, A. (2009). Vygotskian perspectives on using dramatic play to enhance children's development and balance creativity with structure in the early childhood classroom. *Early Child Development and Care, 179*(8), 1041–1054. https://doi.org/10.1080/03004430701731654

Harris, K. I. (2016). Let's play at the park! Family pathways promoting spiritual resources to inspire nature, pretend play, storytelling, intergenerational play and celebrations. *International Journal of Children's Spirituality, 21*(2), 90–103. https://doi.org/10.1080/1364436X.2016.1164669

Heinrichs, J. (2016). The co-creation of a "kinder garden." *Journal of Childhood Studies, 41*(1), 16–23. https://doi.org/10.18357/jcs.v41i1.15694

Hosaka, T., Numata, S., & Koun, S. (2018). Relationship between childhood nature play and adulthood participation in nature-based recreation among urban residents in Tokyo area [Research note]. *Landscape and Urban Planning, 180*, 1–4. https://doi.org/10.1016/j.landurbplan.2018.08.002

Hostettler Scharer, J. (2017). Supporting young children's learning in a dramatic play environment. *Journal of Childhood Studies, 42*(3), 62–69. https://doi.org/10.18357/jcs.v42i3.17895

Houser, N., Roach, L., Stone, M. R., Turner, J., & Kirk, S. F. L. (2016). Let the children play: Scoping review on the implementation and use of loose parts for promoting physical activity participation. *AIMS Public Health, 3*(4), 781–799. https://doi.org/10.3934/publichealth.2016.4.781

International Play Association. (1989). *The child's right to play.* https://ipaworld.org/childs-right-to-play/the-childs-right-to-play/

Izenstark, D., & Ebata, A. T. (2016). Theorizing family-based nature activities and family functioning: The integration of attention restoration theory with a family routines and rituals perspective. *Journal of Family Theory & Review, 8*(2), 137–153. https://doi.org/10.1111/jftr.12138

Izenstark, D., & Ebata, A. T. (2019). Why families go outside: An exploration of mothers' and daughters' family-based nature activities. *Leisure Sciences, 44*(5), 559–577. https://doi.org/10.1080/01490400.2019.1625293

Johnson, J. (2000). *Design for learning: Values, qualities, and processes of enriching school landscapes* (Landscape Architecture Technical Information Series). American Society of Landscape Architects. https://vegetableproject.org/wp-content/uploads/2017/04/Landscape-architects-2000.pdf

Keniger, L. E., Gaston, K. J., Irvine, K. N., & Fuller, R. A. (2013). What are the benefits of interacting with nature? *International Journal of Environmental Research and Public Health, 10*(3), 913–935. https://doi.org/10.3390/ijerph10030913

Khomais, S., Al-Khalidi, N., & Alotaibi, D. (2019). Dramatic play in relation to self-regulation in preschool age. *Contemporary Issues in Education Research (CIER), 12*(4), 103–112. https://doi.org/10.19030/cier.v12i4.10323

Klein, D., Türk, S., & Roth, R. (2018). Outdoor psychomotor activities: Bringing children to nature. *Advances in Physical Education, 8*(2), 1–7. https://doi.org/10.4236/ape.2018.82022

Kutska, K. (2013, August 5). The benefits of risky play. *Playground Professionals.* https://playgroundprofessionals.com/play/benefits-risky-play#:~:text=Risky%20play%20is%20universal%20and,%E2%80%9C

Laaksoharju, T., Rappe, E., & Kaivola, T. (2012). Garden affordances for social learning, play, and for building nature-child relationship. *Urban Forestry & Urban Greening, 11*(2), 195–203. https://doi.org/10.1016/j.ufug.2012.01.003

Lai, N. K., Ang, T. F., Por, L. Y., & Liew, C. S. (2018). The impact of play on child development- a literature review. *European Early Childhood Education Research Journal, 26*(5), 625–643. https://doi.org/10.1080/1350293X.2018.1522479

Lee, E. Y., Bains, A., Hunter, S., Ament, A., Brazo-Sayavera, J., Carson, V., Hakimi, S., Huang, W. Y., Janssen, I., Lee, M., Lim, H., Silva, D. A. S., & Tremblay, M. S. (2021). Systematic review of the correlates of outdoor play and time among children aged 3–12 years. *International Journal of Behavioral Nutrition and Physical Activity, 18*, Article 41. https://doi.org/10.1186/s12966-021-01097-9

Lester, S., & Russell, W. (2010). *Children's right to play: An examination of the importance of play in the lives of children worldwide* (Working Paper No. 57). Bernard van

Leer Foundation. https://issuu.com/bernardvanleerfoundation/docs/childrens_right_to_play_an_examination_of_the_impo/4

Levy, L., & Gottlieb, J. (1984). Learning disabled and non-LD children at play. *Remedial and Special Education, 5*(6), 43–50. https://doi.org/10.1177/074193258400500607

Listokin, J. (2011). Project N.O.I.S.E.E.[sm]: Intergenerational laughter, squeals and giggles. *Journal of Intergenerational Relationships, 9*, 476–480. https://doi.org/10.1080/153507 70.2011.619415

Lohr, V. I., & Pearson-Mims, C. H. (2005). Children's active and passive interactions with plants influence their attitudes towards trees and gardening as adults. *HortTechnology, 15*(3), 472–476. https://doi.org/10.21273/HORTTECH.15.3.0472

Maynard, C. N., Adams, R. A., Lazo-Flores, T., & Warnock, K. (2009). An examination of the effects of teacher intervention during sensory play on the emotional development of preschoolers. *Family & Consumer Sciences Research Journal, 38*(1), 26–35. https://doi.org/10.1111/j.1552-3934.2009.00003.x

McCormick, R. (2017). Does access to green space impact the mental well-being of children: A systematic review. *Journal of Pediatric Nursing, 37*, 3–7. https://doi.org/10.1016/j.pedn.2017.08.027

McFarland, A. L., Zajicek, J. M., & Waliclek, T. M. (2014). The relationship between parental attitudes toward nature and the amount of time children spend in outdoor nature. *Journal of Leisure Research, 46*(5), 525–539. https://doi.org/10.1080/00222216.2014.1 1950341

Mergen, B. (2003). Review essay: Children and nature in history. *Environmental History, 8*(4), 643–668. https://doi.org/10.2307/3985888

Milteer, R. M., & Ginsburg, K. R. (2012). The importance of play in promoting healthy child development and maintaining strong parent–child bond: Focus on children in poverty. *Pediatrics, 129*(1), e204–e213. https://doi.org/10.1542/peds.2011-2953

Miranda, N., Larrea, I., Muela, A., & Barandiaran, A. (2017). Preschool children's social play and involvement in the outdoor environment. *Early Education and Development, 28*(5), 525–540. https://doi.org/10.1080/10409289.2016.1250550

Moore, R. C., Cosco, N., Sherk, J., Bieber, B., Varela, S., Gurina, N., & Murphy, J. (2009). *Creating & retrofitting play environments: Best practice guidelines.* Playcore Inc. and Natural Learning Initiative, College of Design. NC State University. https://www.playcore.com/programs/naturegrounds

National Recreation and Park Association. (n.d.). *About.* https://www.nrpa.org/about-national-recreation-and-park-association/

Neill, P. (2013). Open-ended materials belong outside too! *HighScope, 27*(2), 1–8. https://highscope.org/wp-content/uploads/2018/08/156.pdf

Nicholson, S. (1971). How not to cheat children: The theory of loose parts. *Landscape Architecture, 62*, 30–35.

Nijhof, S. L., Vinkers, C. H., van Geelen, S. M., Duijff, S. N., Achterberg, E. J. M., van der Net, J., Veltkamp, R. C., Grootenhuis, M. A., van de Putte, E. M., Hillegers, M. H. J., van der Brug, A. W., Wierenga, C. J., Benders, M. J. N. L., Engels, R. C. M. E., van der Ent, C. K., Vanderschuren, L. J. M. J., & Lesscher, H. M. B. (2018). Healthy play, better coping: The importance of play for the development of children in health and disease. *Neuroscience & Biobehavioral Reviews, 95*, 421–429. https://doi.org/10.1016/j.neubiorev.2018.09.024

Paggi, M. E., Jopp, D., & Hertzog, C. (2016). The importance of leisure activities in the relationship between physical health and well-being in a life span sample. *Gerontology, 62*, 450–458. https://doi.org/10.1159/000444415

Palmer, A. A., Freeman, P. A., & Zabriski, R. B. (2007). Family deepening: A qualitative inquiry into the experience of families who participate in service expeditions. *Journal of Leisure Research, 39*(3), 438–458. https://doi.org/10.1080/00222216.2007.11950116

Parten, M. B. (1932). Social participation among pre-school children. *Journal of Abnormal and Social Psychology, 27*(3), 243–269. https://doi.org/10.1037/h0074524

Perren, S., Sticca, F., Weiss-Hanselmann, B., & Burkhardt Bossi, C. (2019). Let us play together! Can play tutoring stimulate children's social pretend play level? *Journal of Early Childhood Research, 17*(3), 205–219. https://doi.org/10.1177/1476718X19849248

Preuß, M., Nieuwenhuijsen, M., Marquez, S., Cirach, M., Dadvand, P., Triguero-Mas, M., Gidlow, C., Grazuleviciene, R., Kruize, H., & Zijlema, W. (2019). Low childhood nature exposure is associated with worse mental health in adulthood. *International Journal of Environmental Research and Public Health, 16*(10), Article 1809. https://doi.org/10.3390/ijerph16101809

Robertson, N., Yim, B., & Paatsch, L. (2020) Connections between children's involvement in dramatic play and the quality of early childhood environments. *Early Child Development and Care, 190*(3), 376–389. https://doi.org/10.1080/03004430.2018.1473389

Roopnarine, J. L. (2011). Cultural variations in beliefs about play, parent-child play, and children's play: Meaning for childhood development. In A. D. Pellegrini (Ed.), The Oxford handbook of the development of play (pp. 19–37). Oxford University Press.

Sando, O. J. (2019). The outdoor environment and children's health: A multilevel approach. *International Journal of Play, 8*(1), 39–52. https://doi.org/10.1080/21594937.2019.1580336

Sandseter, E. B. H. (2007). Categorizing risky play: How can we identify risk-taking in children's play? *European Early Childhood Education Research Journal, 5*(2), 237–252. https://doi.org/10.1080/13502930701321733

Sandseter, E. B. H. (2009a). Characteristics of risky play. *Journal of Adventure Education & Outdoor Learning, 9*(1), 3–21. https://doi.org/10.1080/14729670802702762

Sandseter, E. B. H. (2009b). Children's expressions of exhilaration and fear in risky play. *Contemporary Issues in Early Childhood, 10*(2), 92–106. https://doi.org/10.2304/ciec.2009.10.2.92

Sandseter, E. B. H., & Kennair, L. E. O. (2011). Children's risky play from an evolutionary perspective: The anti-phobic effects of thrilling experiences. *Evolutionary Psychology, 9*(2). https://doi.org/10.1177/147470491100900212

Scharer, J. H. (2017). Supporting young children's learning in a dramatic play environment. *Journal of Childhood Studies, 42*(3), 62–69. https://doi.org/10.18357/jcs.v42i3.17895

Siyahhan, S., Barab, S. A., & Downton, M. P. (2010). Using activity theory to understand intergenerational play: The case of family quest. *International Journal of Computer-Supported Collaborative Learning, 5*, 415–432. https://doi.org/10.1007/s11412-010-9097-1

Spence, L., & Radunovich, H. L. (2008). *Developing intergenerational relationships.* University of Florida IFAS Extension, FCS2282 [Course]. https://doi.org/10.32473/edis-fy1007-2007

Stone, M. R., & Faulkner, G. E. J. (2014). Outdoor play in children: Associations with objectively-measured physical activity, sedentary behavior and weight status. *Preventive Medicine, 65*, 122–127. https://doi.org/10.1016/j.ypmed.2014.05.008

Tandon, P. S., Zhou, C., & Christakis, D. A. (2012). Frequency of parent-supervised outdoor play of US preschool-aged children. *Archives of Pediatrics & Adolescent Medicine, 166*(8), 707–712. https://doi.org/10.1001/archpediatrics.2011.1835

Tillmann, S., Tobin, D., Avison, A., & Gilliland, J. (2018). Mental health benefits of interactions with nature in children and teenagers: A systematic review. *Journal of Epidemiology and Community Health, 72*(10), 958–966. https://doi.org/10.1136/jech-2018-210436

Tremblay, M. S., Gray, C., Babcock, S., Barnes, J., Costas Bradstreet, C., Carr, D., Chabot, G., Choquette, L., Chorney, D., Collyer, C., Herrington, S., Janson, K., Janssen, I., Larouche, R., Pickett, W., Power, M. Sanseter. E. B. H., Simon, B., & Brussoni, M. (2015). Position statement on active outdoor play. *International Journal of Environmental Research and Public Health, 12*(6), 6475–6505. https://doi.org/10.3390/ijerph120606475

Tremblay, R. E. (2010). Developmental origins of disruptive behaviour problems: The "original sin" hypothesis, epigenetics, and their consequences for prevention. *Journal of Psychology and Psychiatry, 51*(4), 341–367. https://doi.org/10.1111/j.1469-7610-2010.02211.x

United Nations. (1989). *Convention on the rights of the child.* http://wunrn.org/reference/pdf/Convention_Rights_Child.PDF

van Dijk-Wesselius, J. E., Maas, J., Hovinga, D., van Vugt, M., & van den Berg, A. E. (2018). The impact of greening schoolyards on the appreciation, and physical, cognitive and social-emotional well-being of schoolchildren: A prospective intervention study. *Landscape and Urban Planning, 180*, 15–26. https://doi.org/10.1016/j.landurbplan.2018.08.003

Vygotsky, L. S. (1978). *Mind in society: Development of higher psychological processes.* Harvard University Press.

Wagenfeld, A., Sotelo, M., & Kamp, D. (2019). Designing an impactful sensory garden for children and youth with autism spectrum disorder. *Children, Youth and Environments, 29*(1), 137–152. https://doi.org/10.7721/chilyoutenvi.29.1.0137

Wagenfeld, A., Young, D., & Westley, M. (2014, July 14). Let's ALL play. *OT Practice, 19*(16), 7–11.

Watts, T., Stagnitti, K., & Brown, T. (2014). Relationship between play and sensory processing: A systematic review. *American Journal of Occupational Therapy, 68*(2), e37–e46. https://doi.org/10.5014/ajot.2014.009787

Weisberg, D. S. (2015). Pretend play. *WIREs: Cognitive Science, 6*(3), 249–261. https://doi.org/10.1002/wcs.1341

Wilkes-Gillan, S., Bundy, A., Cordier, R., Lincoln, M., & Chen, Y.-W. (2016). A randomised controlled trial of a play-based intervention to improve the social play skills of children with attention deficit hyperactivity disorder (ADHD). *PLoS ONE, 11*(8), Article e0160558. https://doi.org/10.1371/journal.pone.0160558

Yang, C., & Jia Wang, S. (2017). Sandtime: A tangible interaction featured sensory play installation for children to increase social connection. *EAI Endorsed Transactions on Creative Technologies, 4*(10), Article e4. https://doi.org/10.4108/eai.4-9-2017.153056

Yogman, M., Garner, A., Hutchinson, J., Hirsh-Pasek, K., Golinkoff, R. M., & Committee on Psychosocial Aspects of Child and Family Health, & Council on Communications and Media. (2018). The power of play: A pediatric role in enhancing development in young children. *Pediatrics, 142*(3), Article e20182058. https://doi.org/10.1542/peds.2018-2058

Yule, K., Houston, J., & Grych, J. (2019). Resilience in children exposed to violence: A meta-analysis of protective factors across ecological contexts. *Clinical Child and Family Psychology Review, 22*, 406–431. https://doi.org/10.1007/s10567-019-00293-1

4

TYPICAL CHILDHOOD DEVELOPMENT

Years ago, Amy taught life span developmental psychology at a small suburban college. On the first day of the infant and child course, she always told her students that this was going to be the most important class they would take in college. Lots of eye rolls and giggles ensued. However, by the end of the semester, the students wholeheartedly acknowledged that the period of infant and childhood development is critical in laying the foundation for the trajectory toward adulthood. What was Amy's justification for such a provocative statement, and what exactly is development?

Introduction

According to the ICF (WHO, 2007), *development* is a "dynamic process by which the child moves progressively from dependency on others for all activities in infancy towards physical, social and psychological maturity and independence in adolescence" (p. 16). As a dynamic process, all body systems—such as the digestive, immune, circulatory, metabolic, and nervous systems—work together. They also work independently of each other to take in information, make sense of it, and adapt to it for better or for worse (Harvard Center on the Developing Child, 2020).

How children experience and respond to this information helps shape the adults they will become. Children grow and develop within physical and social *contexts* or *environments* (we use the terms interchangeably). The caregiving the children receive, the experiences they have, and the culture in which they are raised mediate these contexts (Bornstein et al., 2012). Environmental factors influencing children's ability to participate and engage are the "physical, social and attitudinal environment in which people live and conduct their lives" (WHO, 2007, p. 16). The quality and quantity of opportunities provided early to children to grow, develop, and thrive lay the foundation for everything else in their lives. In short, the

DOI: 10.4324/9781003193890-4

social and physical environmental affordances and opportunities experienced as infants and young children shape lifelong health and well-being. We cannot stress the importance of positive early childhood experiences enough.

These early years of life are when the brain's architecture is under (mega)construction, guided by a complex web of connections between genes, environmental and social-emotional experiences, and the children's behavioral patterns (Walker et al., 2011). Throughout childhood, as children grow and develop on their road to independence, so do their environments (WHO, 2007). In other words, a person's inner biology, like their genes; outside influences, such as nutrition, environmental conditions, caregiver nurturing; and how the person responds to these influences are the building blocks for future physical, social-emotional, and cognitive development (Bornstein et al., 2012). Genetics cannot be changed, but the ways caregivers nurture children and the experiences children have or are exposed to play an enormously important role in how children develop. Although their brains remain plastic and able to adapt and respond to the social (relationships they have) and physical (places they are) environmental events experienced in the home and community throughout their lives, never are they more sensitive to these experiences than in the first 5 years of life. Once again, what happens early on dictates the entire course of a child's life.

In this chapter, we focus on typical childhood development. The three areas we explore are physical, social-emotional, and cognitive (including language) development. We look at what it means to develop, the ways developmental scholars explain how children develop, and why all children must be provided with the best possible resources to grow, thrive, and become their best selves. This is important information, particularly when creating all types of play spaces for children because making the right choices matters. Along with the chapter's text, a key feature is a developmental milestones chart (Table 4.2) to help guide you in making age-appropriate design decisions when creating inclusive outdoor play spaces for children and their families.

Developmental Periods

There are five periods or stages of child development: prenatal, infancy, early childhood, middle childhood, and adolescence (Berk, 2018a, 2018b; Shaffer, 2013). In a typically developing child, these stages progress as described in this section, beginning in the prenatal stage until adolescence.

Prenatal

The prenatal period is the time from conception until birth. A baby is considered full term if born between 37 and 41 weeks of gestation. In the United States, a full-term baby's average length and weight are 20 inches and 7.5 pounds. During the prenatal period, the fetus is very sensitive to environmental influences, such as exposure to toxins, maternal stress, and nutrition, while growing faster than at any other time in life.

Infancy

The infancy period begins at birth and lasts until about 15–18 months. Like the prenatal period, infancy is a period of rapid growth. Within the first 18 months, typically developing infants will learn to walk, talk, feed themselves, and relate to their social and physical environments. During infancy, children learn about their world through sensorimotor experiences.

Early Childhood

The *early childhood* period begins at 18 months and lasts until about age 6 years. Early childhood is characterized by social-emotional development and an explosion in cognitive development, particularly with understanding and speaking language. In early childhood, young children begin to develop relationships with peers and experience a bit of independence from their primary caregivers as they attend preschool and primary school.

Middle Childhood

The middle childhood *period* starts at 6 years and ends at about 12 years, with the onset of adolescence. During middle childhood, children begin to focus on academics while refining gross (large muscle, like sports) and fine (small muscle, like writing) motor and social-emotional skills, particularly peer relationships.

Adolescence

The period of adolescence begins at about 12 years and ends at age 18 years. It is during adolescence that children experience significant social-emotional and physical changes as they prepare for adulthood. Sometimes considered a period of intense turmoil, the tasks of adolescence include addressing self-identity and establishing autonomy as adolescents prepare for adulthood.

Developmental Theory

Even though developmental scholars differ in their explanations of how typical development happens, it mostly occurs the same way and at the same time for every child. It is important to understand that many factors can derail—or at least significantly affect—typical development. This list of roadblocks to healthy development includes poverty, poor nutrition, caregiver mental health issues, violence, disease, and genetic factors.

There are two overarching explanations for the childhood developmental trajectory: continuity and discontinuity. *Continuity* theorists believe that development occurs as a process of accumulation, in a gradual, continual process. For instance, children become more skilled at walking or talking in the same way they gain weight—slowly and gradually. *Discontinuity* theorists view development in a stepwise, distinct sequence. Walking happens in a sequential fashion. Each motor milestone from the infant first holding their head up when placed on their belly leads to the skills they need to be upright and take those first steps at about 12–18 months. The same stepwise sequence applies to talking: The baby coos, babbles, and then says their first words. Continuity and discontinuity theorists share the understanding that children become more skillful and increasingly ready to undertake new experiences and challenges as they develop. Note that this chapter's milestone chart (Table 4.2) represents more of a discontinuity, stepwise developmental model.

Viewing development as active or passive is another crucial concept to explore. The idea that children are the primary determiner of their abilities aligns with an *active* view of development. A *passive* view suggests that outside influences, such as physical environmental and social experiences and biological characteristics beyond the child's control shape whom the child will become.

Finally, let's explore the nature-versus-nurture development debate. The *nature* view suggests that development occurs as it does because of each child's inner biology and genetics. *Nurture*, on the other hand, suggests that children develop as they do based on their physical environmental and social experiences. Most developmental theorists have come to the middle-ground view that a combination of nature and nurture shapes how children develop.

Developmental Theorists and Their Theories

It is beyond the scope of this chapter to provide more than a brief overview of several influential developmental theorists and their theories. Nevertheless, the interested reader is encouraged to study further the theories that spark their curiosity. Table 4.1 provides information about developmental theories and how they relate to play. Take a few moments to reflect on the theories that most apply to your design, planning, educational, or therapeutic philosophy. If you feel that selecting one is too limiting, you are not alone. Many people find wisdom in several developmental theories and struggle to select just one that aligns with their work.

The Developmental March

Development does not happen in a vacuum, nor does each area of development proceed in isolation (Denham et al., 2009). All childhood development aspects—physical, social-emotional, and cognitive—are interconnected and influenced by the environmental contexts in which children spend their days (Bronfenbrenner & Morris, 1998). These environments could be their homes, childcare centers, schools, houses of worship, parks and play spaces, neighborhoods, medical and dental offices, museums, or shops, to name a few. What happens in each context can influence engagement in other contexts (e.g., experiencing bullying in a play space could affect how a child engages at school) and have a lasting impact on development.

Cross-culturally and throughout the world, when biological/genetic, environmental, and social circumstances enable typical development to unfold, its progression follows pretty much the same course. Think of achieving developmental milestones as an unfolding and unfurling process. Developmental *norms* are the

TABLE 4.1 Developmental Theories and Play

Theorist	Overview	Relationship to play
Jean Piaget (1896–1980)	Development proceeds sequentially and is guided by internal processes (Piaget & Inhelder, 1969).	Play as hard as you can, get into it, get dirty, and then play some more. Children thrive when they have many hands-on and observational experiences to help them learn about the world.
Lev Vygotsky (1896–1934)	Given the time they need, children learn through social experiences and with support from others who are more experienced (Vygotsky, 1978).	Keep trying and working harder. Skills develop a bit at a time by increasingly challenging, hands-on play activities with help from others.
Sigmund Freud (1856–1939)	Personality develops on its own and is also influenced by emotions.	Messy and creative play is great. It helps nurture development.
Erik Erikson (1902–1994)	Becoming a well-adjusted or maladapted adult depends on how one accomplishes specific tasks in a life-span developmental sequence (Erikson, 1963, 1982).	Structure play to be rewarding. Play needs to be a positive experience that supports autonomy, resilience, and growth.
Abraham Maslow (1908–1979)	Navigating through the hierarchy of needs can motivate someone to become their most self-fulfilled person (Maslow, 1968, 1970).	Where play happens matters. A safe place to play must be provided before play materials and elements can be used, enjoyed, and a source of satisfaction.
Urie Bronfenbrenner (1917–2005)	A child's social-emotional and physical environments (ecosystem) highly influence development (Bronfenbrenner, 1979, 1986).	It's all about place. Design, modify, or adapt play spaces so they are inclusive for all.
B. F. Skinner (1904–1990)	Humans develop through learning that shapes behaviors. Learning is a change in behavior that results from experiences.	Encourage and reinforce play. Support positive play behaviors by providing many choices and options to learn new skills.
Albert Bandura (1925–2021)	Cognition develops because of observation and modeling others' behaviors and actions.	Play together. Social play enables children to watch and learn from peers.
Konrad Lorenz (1903–1989)	What happens emotionally or physically in critical or sensitive developmental periods can make or break future healthy development.	Choose play elements wisely. The quality of play materials matters and can support or impede development.

Modified from: Wagenfeld (2017).

age ranges during which milestones typically occur. Although the typical and sequential development patterns are not always textbook perfect—humans are not
programmable machines who reach their milestones at the same time—infants bab-
ble and coo before they say their highly anticipated first word. They roll before
they sit, they use their whole hand to grasp a toy before they pick up a tiny morsel
of food with their thumb and index finger, and they play alone before discovering
the joys (and challenges!) of playing with peers. Each stage of development, be it
motor, social-emotional, or cognitive, leads to the next more complex level, with
the goal of becoming a fully functional adult. Let's look at how these fascinating
processes occur, beginning with motor development.

Motor Development

Motor development is also referred to as *physical development* because it involves
the body and movement. Typically, motor development happens in a *cephalocaudal* (head-to-toe) pattern. This means that babies' earliest purposeful movements
start at the head and work their way down to the toes. Think about it. When a very
young baby is placed on its belly, it will try and eventually succeed in lifting its
head against gravity. This is momentous! Not long after developing more control
of their head and neck movements, they turn their head from side to side. Then
they raise it higher, so their chest begins to lift off the ground. This head-to-toe development pattern continues as the trunk and spine grow stronger and babies gain
the postural control necessary to develop increasingly complex gross-motor movements like rolling and sitting. Box 4.1 provides a quick overview of cephalocaudal
development. As you look at the list, try to envision how this pattern of gross-motor
development indeed proceeds from head to toe.

**BOX 4.1 TYPICAL CEPHALOCAUDAL DEVELOPMENT
SEQUENCE**

Lifts head slightly when placed on belly
Lift head higher to clear the floor and turns it from side to side
Rolls to side
Rolls from front to back
Rolls from back to front
Sits with support
Sits independently
Gets into hands-and-knees position and rocks back and forth
Begins to creep on all fours (often backwards at first)
Pulls to a stand
Sidesteps along furniture, holding on to it for support
Stands independently
First steps

Another pattern of typical motor development is *proximal to distal*, or closest to furthest from the centerline of the body. The shoulder muscles and joints, closest (proximal) to the chest, are large. They provide support and stability to the elbow and wrist, in turn, supporting the fingers. The base of the fingers near the palm is more stable than are the fingertips, which are farther away (distal). The same pattern holds for the legs. The pelvic/hip muscles and joints help us sit and stand (proximal); the knee supports the ankle, and so on, to the toes (distal).

Proximal control develops before distal control. Babies sit before they get onto all fours and begin to creep. Without proximal shoulder and hip control, babies cannot support themselves on their hands and knees. They cannot begin to move, one arm at a time, with elbows and wrists, which are more distal from the body center than the shoulders, bending and straightening with palms on the floor as they navigate the world.

Let's pause with a nature-related example of the relationship between proximal and distal control. Shoulder stability is important when harvesting tomatoes. Mental map this activity—picking a tomato from the vine. What is the first thing you did when pretending to pluck this juicy, ripe tomato from the vine? Did you "fix" your shoulders and tighten them a bit so you could reach out with one arm and hand to gently grasp the stem while your other hand and fingers popped the tomato off the stem? Try it again without allowing your shoulders to stay fixed and stable. Is it harder to pick your imaginary tomato?

Try another mental mapping activity, this time with your legs. A soccer ball is passed to you, and your job is to kick it to the goal. You need to shore up and tighten your hip and pelvic muscles in your kicking leg, preparing to bend the knee and ankle to contact the ball and get it right into the goal. Do it again, but this time, let your hip feel limp. Now, how easily can your knee and ankle be properly positioned and ready to kick the ball? How hard is it to even stand upright? Although development typically proceeds in a proximal-to-distal fashion, it is essential to understand that some children with limited proximal movement due to genetic or other orthopedic conditions develop distal skills first.

Motor skills are divided into two categories—gross and fine—with the proximal–distal patterns of development factoring into both. As a quick review, *gross* motor skills are the large movements done with the arms or legs. Examples are running, jumping, throwing, or kicking a ball. *Fine* motor skills involve precise hand and finger movements, such as drawing, typing, and buttoning. Typically, gross-motor skills develop before and support fine-motor skills because they require the body's large muscles to initiate the work. We use gross- and fine-motor skills throughout the day—to dress, bathe, feed ourselves, work, and play. Please see Table 4.2 for a comprehensive chart of developmental motor milestones.

Play, Nature, and Motor Development

Motor skills are enhanced and challenged when play happens in nature because there is a higher level of unpredictability when playing outside. Grassy fields are

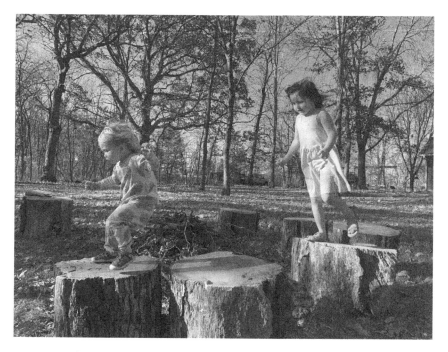

FIGURE 4.1   Gross motor skills are enriched by nature. Credit- Julie Stevens.

uneven compared to indoor flooring; there are boulders to scale, nooks and cran-
nies to explore, and flowers that need to be deadheaded. Some of these elements
require squatting; others require reaching high overhead or to the side. Because
nothing in nature is ever static, children need to bend, stretch, reach, carry, and
above all, *move* to adjust to constantly changing terrain, traverse over (or through)
puddles, and build forts and fairy houses (see Figure 4.1).

Social-Emotional Development

Social-emotional health is foundational to early child development. It has been
linked to cognitive outcomes and later academic performance (Durlak et al., 2011).
For instance, there is a strong connection between early social-emotional development and the later development of complex cognitive functioning and school
readiness (Shonkoff & Phillips, 2000). Five dimensions of social-emotional development lay the foundation for optimal or suboptimal outcomes for children and
the adults they will become (Denham et al., 2009, p. i37): (1) social competence,
(2) attachment, (3) emotional competence, (4) self-perceived competence, and (5)
temperament/personality.

Briefly, *social competence* is effective, developmentally appropriate social interactions with peers and adults. *Attachment* is the profoundly meaningful connection an infant makes with their primary caregiver in the first few years of

TABLE 4.2 Typical Sequence of Developmental Milestones

Age range		Context		
Typically, and in this order, a child will . . .	Motor	Sensory motor/play	Social-emotional	Cognitive/Language
• between birth and 6 months (baby) . . .	• Grasp reflexively • Lift head 45° when on belly • Turn from side to back • Begin to bat at objects • Release objects unintentionally • Reach for and grasp objects • Hold rattle with one or both hands • Bring hands together at midline • Roll from back to front • Balance head steadily when getting help to sit • Begin to move by rocking, rolling, twisting • Bring feet to mouth to suck toes • Grasp object with entire hand and explore it • Begin to let go and move objects from hand to hand • Roll from front to back and back to front • Balance on own in ring sitting	• Be awake 1 of every 10 hours • Startle spontaneously • Alert to sounds • Be soothed by music • Slowly follow objects with eyes • Self-soothe by sucking hand/fingers or pacifier • Look at hands • Explore face, eyes, and mouth with hands • Look for source of sounds • Begin exploratory and interactive play • Follow objects with eyes in a 180° plane • Be responsive for more than an hour at a time • Focus eyes at different distances and see in full color • Follow moving object with eyes	• Demonstrate primary emotions: fear, anger, joy, sadness, disgust, contempt, surprise • Make eye contact if within 18 inches of another person • Learn that crying leads to being picked up (communication begins) • Be interested in people • Smile at human faces • Recognize primary caregivers • Actively seek caregiver's attention • Demonstrate temperament style and activity levels • Start to smile at self in mirror but does not understand it is them • Respond to familiar people • Laugh with others	• Make random sounds • Start to discriminate sounds (speech and other sounds) • Coo or hum to music • Vocalize more and begin to imitate sounds • Study objects for a long time and be very attentive • Turn to source when name is called • Start to entertain self for short periods • Demonstrate increased memory for people, places, and objects • Form perceptual categories based on objects and similar features • Attend to caregiver, who labels objects and events • Make v, th, f, s, sh, m, n, b sounds

(Continued)

TABLE 4.2 (Continued)

Age range	Context			
Typically, and in this order, a child will . . .	*Motor*	*Sensory motor/play*	*Social-emotional*	*Cognitive/Language*
	• Crawl by pulling stomach with legs and steering with arms • Pull objects of interest toward them • Transfer objects from one hand to the other • Reach for toys with one or both hands	• Explore objects with mouth • Experience early signs of depth perception • Hear more accurately • Recognize sounds of native language • Follow path of falling objects • Show sign of sleep patterns emerging; days and nights are usually in sync	• Clearly recognize caregivers and siblings • Try to make contact with others through smiles and vocalizations • Express displeasure • Match adults' emotional expressions during face-to-face interactions • Understand the word "no" • Develop subjective sense of self • Begin to demonstrate a sense of humor	
• between 7 and 12 months (baby) . . .	• Push up on hands and knees and rock back and forth • Begin to creep on all fours • Bounce on feet when held in standing position • Sit independently • Assist in pull to stand from sitting • Creep on hands and knees forward and backward	• Explore body with mouth and hands • Enjoy social games like peek-a-boo • Play vigorously with noisy toys • Hold an object in one hand and simultaneously play with a different toy in the other hand	• Demonstrating primary emotions (anger, fear, sadness) becomes more evident and increases in frequency and intensity • Show interest in being part of social interactions • Become wary of strangers	• Imitate a wide variety of sounds • Imitate hand movements • Look to where others are pointing • Start simple problem-solving • Engage in intentional or goal-directed behavior

(*Continued*)

TABLE 4.2 (Continued)

Age range	Context			
Typically, and in this order, a child will . . .	Motor	Sensory motor/play	Social-emotional	Cognitive/Language
	• Creep while holding an object in one hand • Attempt to grasp objects using a scooping hand motion • Hold two objects in one hand simultaneously • When holding objects in each hand, may hit them together • Clap • Develop a lateral pinch (thumb and side of index finger) pattern • Pick up a string • Creep quickly and efficiently • Begin to right themselves when tipping side to side and backwards in sitting • Begin to take steps with hands held • Stand with hands on furniture • Start to half-kneel (one knee up, the other on the floor) • Pull up to stand • Cruise along furniture • Squat and stoop	• Begin to actively explore the world beyond the door—becoming an explorer • Choose favorite toys to play with • Fear heights and be afraid of vertical surfaces • Focus for about 5 minutes to play alone or with an adult • Enjoy water play • Use fingers versus whole hand to poke and touch objects in play	• Firmly attach to primary caregiver (usually mother) • Object to being confined (e.g., in pram, highchair, crib) • Demonstrate that their sense of humor is developing • Shout for attention • Push away undesirable things (like food!) • Show high levels of separation anxiety • Begin to demonstrate empathy and may cry when another baby cries in their presence • Perform for attention • Seek attention and companionship • Not always cooperative; beginning sense of autonomy	• Understand that even when something is out of sight, it still exists (object permanence) • Imitate simple motor behaviors • Babble • Imitate nonspeech sounds • Imitate consonant/vowel combinations • Begin to use gestures • Understand and obey some words and commands • Wave bye-bye • Display improved memory skills • Work on figuring out simple relationships (such as how a button turns on a toy) • Look at familiar objects and persons when named • Say first meaningful words

(Continued)

TABLE 4.2 (Continued)

Age range			Context	
Typically, and in this order, a child will . . .	Motor	Sensory motor/play	Social-emotional	Cognitive/Language
	• Walk with one hand being held			
	• Crawl up stairs			
	• Pick up small objects with flattened thumb and finger			
	• Purposely release objects			
	• Bang objects together or singularly			
	• Use a thumb, index-, and middle-finger grasp rather than entire hand to pick up objects			
	• Remove objects from containers with one hand			
	• Pick up tiny objects using flattened tip of thumb and flattened tip of index finger			
	• Take lids (if ajar) off boxes			
	• Turn pages of book (not exactly one at a time)			
	• Point			

(Continued)

TABLE 4.2 (Continued)

Age range	Context			
Typically, and in this order, a child will . . .	Motor	Sensory motor/play	Social-emotional	Cognitive/Language
• between 12 and 18 months (baby) . . .	• Stand alone • Lower self to sit from stand • Take first steps using a wide-based stance • Crawl up and down stairs (needs to be taught to descend going backwards) • Roll ball in imitation • Grasp objects using the tip of the thumb and index finger • Put objects in and remove them from containers and boxes • Stack rings on sticks • Open and close things • Walk forward and backward • Walk with stable stops and starts • Walk up and down steps holding a railing or with assist from an adult • Begin to run • Climb on furniture	• Begin to engage in pretend play; use a spoon to feed a baby doll • Enjoy squeezing, twisting, pulling different textured objects • Possibly begin to engage in pretend play; toothbrush becomes a magic wand	• Begin to look to caregiver to gauge own emotional response • Begin to care for dolls or stuffed toys • Start to identify body parts • Imitate gestures and facial expressions • Resist napping and may throw tantrums • Become interested in looking at self in mirror	• Identify animals in pictures when asked • Have a two- to three-word vocabulary (at 12 months) • Complete simple foamboard puzzles • Follow one-step directions • Point to body parts upon request • Have a 10- to 12-word vocabulary and accompanying gestures to communicate thoughts (at 15 months) • Use holographic speech: One word (and accompanying emotions) conveys an entire thought

(Continued)

TABLE 4.2 (Continued)

Age range	Context		
Typically, and in this order, a child will . . .	Motor	Sensory motor/play	Social-emotional	Cognitive/Language
	• Use and reach with preferred hand (hand dominance not yet established) • Build a four-block tower • Put small objects in and remove them from a narrow-necked bottle • Make spontaneous marks with crayons			
• between 18 and 24 months (toddler) . . .	• Walk with stable gait • Sit by self in small chair • Throw ball • Move small objects from fingers to palm of same hand • Place pegs in holes • Put objects into small cups or containers • Scribble using a fisted-hand grasp	• Begin to accept more types of touch, such as roughhousing • Tolerate different clothing textures • Begin to engage in symbolic play, substituting one object for another • Begin to engage in parallel play (playing next to but not with other children) • Play alone or with others for 15 minutes	• Sense of self emerges • Display wider range of emotions • Consistently recognize self in mirror • Show attachment and nurturance toward a stuffed toy	• Know most, if not all, body parts • Follow two-step commands • Hum

(*Continued*)

TABLE 4.2 (Continued)

Age range	Context			
Typically, and in this order; a child will . . .	Motor	Sensory motor/play	Social-emotional	Cognitive/Language
• between 2 and 3 years (toddler) . . .	• Walk up and down stairs independently • Start to run, jump, hop, throw, and catch balls • As balance improves, demonstrate more coordinated walking patterns • Run proficiently • Catch large ball with hands and arms • Throw ball • Walk up several stairs using alternating feet pattern • Tiptoe • Walk backward • Kick ball • Build an eight-block tower • Open loose jar lids • Begin to use scissors • Imitate someone drawing vertical lines on paper • Draw circles	• Independently select toys • Play house and imitate domestic tasks • Become less dependent on realistic toys • Engage in more complex pretend play	• Begin developing coping strategies • Seek caregiver approval • Become less self-centered • Show signs of improved self-concept and self-esteem • Demonstrate cooperation and instrumental aggression (aggressive act done on purpose to achieve an outcome) • Understand causes and consequences of basic emotions • Demonstrate increased empathy • Frequently imitate caregiver behavior • Begin to be aware of gender identity	• Has a 220-word vocabulary • Utter three-word sentences • Use personal pronoun "I" • Refer to self by name • Begin to ask questions • Begin to sort objects by shape and color • Find hidden objects embedded in sand or other medium • Demonstrate simple perspective-taking • Rapidly acquire new words • Use sentences that start to follow basic word order of native language • Display effective conversational skills, such as turn-taking and staying on topic

(Continued)

TABLE 4.2 (Continued)

Age range	Motor	Context		
Typically, and in this order, a child will . . .		Sensory motor/play	Social-emotional	Cognitive/Language
	• Screw and unscrew 3-inch lids from jars • String 1-inch beads • Begin to show signs of hand dominance • Move small objects from palm to fingers within same hand		• Recognize self in a photo	• Begin to use telegraphic speech—short sentences that contain only essential words "girl juice" may mean "I want some juice" • Increase use of pronouns • Ask "why?" • Understand simple questions • Name objects in a picture • Match and discriminate colors • Complete simple two-piece puzzles
• between 3 and 4 years (preschooler) . . .	• Stand on one foot • Jump in place • Pedal tricycle • Demonstrate more coordinated running, hopping, throwing, catching skills • Begin to gallop and one-foot skipping • Build 10-block tower • Construct three- to four-block train	• Begin to participate in more complex exploratory and imitative play • Demonstrate more imaginative and creative play scenarios • Begin turn-taking in play	• Begin to understand different emotional responses • Regulate emotions better • Become better at emotional self-regulation • Demonstrate more self-conscious emotions	• Assemble 8- to 10-piece puzzle • Have a 900- to 1,000-word vocabulary • Speak in short (four+ words) sentences • Use plurals and tenses (not always correctly) • Master increasingly complex grammatical structures

(Continued)

TABLE 4.2 (Continued)

Age range	Context		
Typically, and in this order, a child will . . .	Motor	Sensory motor/play	Social-emotional	Cognitive/Language
	• String half-inch beads • Fold a piece of paper • Snip with scissors • Use a shoulder-generated two-finger grasp of a pencil, marker, or crayon • Copy vertical and horizontal lines, circles, square, and cross • Draw a picture of a person—head with legs		• Display humorous and mischievous behaviors • Be negative and oppositional at times • Form first friendships • Distinguish moral rules from conventions • Show preference for same-sex playmates	• Occasionally overextend grammatical rules to exceptions • Use private speech to guide behavior in challenging tasks • Demonstrate ability to count to 10 by rote with no one-to-one correspondence (not touching a series of objects while counting) • Tell simple stories • Use language more than actions to communicate • Follow two-step directions • Recognize simple shapes • Demonstrate more sustained and planned attention • Count a small number of objects • Tell difference between letters, numbers, and nonwriting (e.g., shapes)

TABLE 4.2 (Continued)

Age range		Context		
Typically, and in this order, a child will . . .	Motor	Sensory motor/play	Social-emotional	Cognitive/Language
• between 4 and 6 years (child) . . .	• Descend steps with alternating-gait pattern • Balance on one foot • Hop and skip • Catch ball using hands • Bounce a ball • Throw overhand • Cut straight and simple curved lines with 25% accuracy • Begin to use tools such as hammers • Perform rapid, alternating forearm movements (e.g., beating a drum) • Copy triangle, simple words, and name with limited awareness of spacing or size • Draw more elaborate figures; write names	• Display pretend play that is more logical • Engage in more cooperative play	• Begin to mask emotions • Resolve conflicts with peers with greater ease • Demonstrate guilt • Show increased peer interaction • Show improved ability to interpret, predict, and influence others' emotional reactions • Rely more on language vs. actions to express empathy • Have acquired many morally relevant rules and behaviors • Demonstrate racial identity • Engage in gender-stereotyped beliefs and behavior	• Repeat a 5- to 10-word sentence • Repeat five to seven numbers • Carry on a reciprocal conversation • Begin to think more logically • Begin to demonstrate cause-and-effect thinking • Understand "why" questions • Begin to understand opposites, such as big and little • Understand differences, such as circle and square • Demonstrate one-to-one correspondence with counting three objects • Have a vocabulary of about 10,000 words • Show mastery of many complex grammatical forms

(Continued)

TABLE 4.2 (Continued)

Age range	Context			
Typically, and in this order, a child will . . .	Motor	Sensory motor/play	Social-emotional	Cognitive/Language
• between 6 and 9 years (child) . . .	• Master ball skills • Master bike-riding (6–7 years) • Learn to swim • Learn to skate • Demonstrate faster, more coordinated running, jumping, throwing, catching, kicking, batting, dribbling • Become adept at using school tools (pencil, scissors, glue, keyboard) • Learn and master manuscript writing • Writing becomes smaller and more legible • Letter reversals decline • Learn and master cursive writing • Drawings become more organized and detailed; include some depth cues • Drawing becomes increasingly more representational	• Engage in more ritualized, dramatic, pretend play • Engage in formal games as a form of play • Become interested in collections and hobbies • Commonly engage in games with rules	• Begin to understand other people's views • Show improved ability to comply with display rules of emotions • Demonstrate improved sense of self • Further develop self-esteem • Recognize own strengths and limitations • Use psychological traits to define self • Begin to engage in more like-gender social relationships • Recognize that people may experience more than one emotion at a time • Become increasingly more responsible and independent	• Create more representational drawings • Show emergence of reverse thinking; analyze from end, then back to beginning • Demonstrate improved perception of reality • Understand cause and effect • Have a well-formed memory • Demonstrate early executive-processing skills, improved problem-solving, better focus and attention to task • Apply logic to thinking • Show a greater understanding of spatial concepts • Give clear, well-organized directions

(Continued)

TABLE 4.2 (Continued)

Age range		Context		
Typically, and in this order, a child will . . .	Motor	Sensory motor/play	Social-emotional	Cognitive/Language
			• Demonstrate more prosocial peer interaction; decline in physical aggression toward peers	• Demonstrate attention that is more selective, adaptable, and planful
			• Self-esteem and sense of mastery tend to increase	• Use memory strategies of rehearsal and organization
			• Use adaptive set of strategies to regulate emotions	• Word definitions are concrete, referring to functions and appearance
			• Become better at "stepping into another's shoes" and viewing self from other person's perspective	• Use memory strategies such as rehearsal and organization more effectively
			• Begin to form peer groups	• Begin to elaborate in speech
			• Become aware of more gender stereotypes, including personality traits and school subjects; has a more flexible appreciation of what males and females can do	• Use more complex grammatical construction in speech and writing
			• Show increased in sibling rivalry	• Demonstrate conversational strategies that are more refined
				• Apply multiple memory strategies simultaneously

(Continued)

TABLE 4.2 (Continued)

Age range	Context			
Typically, and in this order, a child will . . .	Motor	Sensory motor/play	Social-emotional	Cognitive/Language
• between 10 and 18 years (pre-adolescent/adolescent) . . .	• Become proficient with all gross-motor tasks • Become proficient at all fine-motor skills and apply this ability to all aspects of life, including school, work, self-care, health management, and leisure activities	• Participate in competitive team sports	• Define their identity • Make a shift so that self-concept becomes refined and based on other people's perspectives • In a quest for autonomy, may bring strife into caregiver–child relationship • Grapple with issues of sexuality • Begin to date • Demonstrate increased moodiness and caregiver–child conflict • Spend less time with caregivers and siblings • Spend more time with peers	• Think hypothetically and abstractly • Become more proficient with verbal and mathematical skills • Experience a sense of invulnerability ("it can't happen to me"); may be problematic and danger-provoking • Become capable of formal operational reasoning • Become better at coordinating theory with evidence • Argue more effectively • Become more self-conscious and self-focused

(Continued)

TABLE 4.2 (Continued)

Age range		Context		
Typically, and in this order, a child will . . .	Motor	Sensory motor/play	Social-emotional	Cognitive/Language
			• Engage in friendships based on intimacy and loyalty • Engage in cliques with peers with similar values that unite and form crowds • Demonstrate increased conformity to peer pressure • Demonstrate increased self-esteem • Likely searching for an identity • Importance of cliques and crowd declines • Probably start dating	• Become more idealistic and critical • Become less self-conscious and self-focused • Become better at everyday planning and decision-making

Modified from: Wagenfeld et al. (2017). Compiled from Berk (2018a, 2018b), Berger (2019), Bowlby (1988), Craig and Baucum (2002), Davies (1999), Dunn and Craig (2006), Emde et al. (1976), Erhardt (1982), Feldman (2016), Jacobs and Jacobs (2014), Kagan (1984), Kit et al. (2017), Logigan and Ward (1989), Piaget and Inhelder (1969), Rapee et al. (2019), Santrock (2018), Shaffer (2013), Steinberg et al. (2010), Stern (1985), Velikonjia et al. (2017), and VORT Corporation (2010).

life. The quality of this first attachment sets the stage for all future relationships throughout life. *Emotional competence* is the ability to be aware of one's own and others' emotions, act upon them, self-regulate emotional responses, and engage in interpersonal communication. *Self-perceived competence* increases in complexity with age and experience. It is a self-evaluation of one's cognitive, social, and physical abilities, particularly compared to others. *Temperament/personality* refers to differences in self-regulation and emotional reactivity, which is understood to have a genetic basis (Denham et al., 2009, pp. i38–i45) (see Figure 4.2).

The quality of the interactions with adults and other children affects social-emotional development positively or negatively (Laaksoharju et al., 2012). Supportive and nurturing interaction is affirming for children and positively influences social-emotional development. On the other hand, there is a strong connection between growing up in poverty, having a parent (particularly a mother) or caregiver with mental health issues, or having a trauma history and childhood social-emotional vulnerabilities. Children who experience these daunting adversities are more susceptible to chronic mental and physical illnesses (Folger et al., 2017) than children who do not face these obstacles to healthy development. For instance, exposure to adverse childhood experiences (ACEs) such as trauma, violence, caregiver incarceration, poverty, and homelessness early in life makes children highly

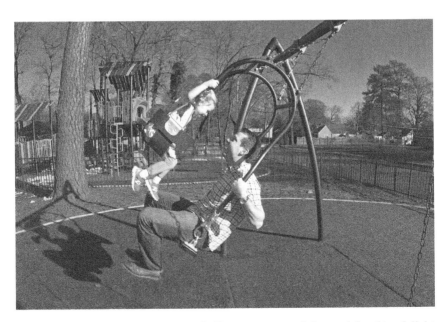

FIGURE 4.2   A spontaneous moment of affect attunement; father and daughter delighting in the shared experience of swinging. Credit- GameTime, a PlayCore Company.

vulnerable to stress and social-emotional challenges. (Please refer to Chapter 6, "Inclusive Design," for more detailed information about ACEs.)

Poor social-emotional development in childhood has a cascading negative impact on behavior, academic achievement, and physical problems (Treat et al., 2020). Excessive exposure to stress during childhood can put a child on constant high alert, which is detrimental to learning. It is nearly impossible for a child in a highly reactive emotional state to focus on what is important in the classroom at any given moment. Stress in childhood can also have lasting negative physical impacts, such as cancer, cardiovascular and digestive issues, and diabetes in adulthood.

According to Blalock et al. (2019), "children's social-emotional competencies are related to their ability to succeed and thrive" (p. 239). Children who do not struggle with social-emotional challenges tend to demonstrate better behavior and in-class performance, get along better with peers and adults, and have a lower risk for mental health issues than children with such issues (Durlak et al., 2011). Children who are stressed are more likely than their peers who report lower personal- and school-related stresses to struggle in school (Li & Sullivan, 2016). Lacking strong social-emotional competency puts children at risk for learning and physical challenges during childhood and later in life.

Play, Nature, and Social-Emotional Development

Nature boosts mental health: Exposure to or contact with greened environments positively influences mental health (Dettweiler et al., 2017). First, let's clarify that *green* does not mean just the color. Green in this situation means an association with nature, such as waterways, forests, parks, play spaces, farms, and gardens. For children, nearby nature is a buffer for sound mental health and resilience (Wells & Evans, 2003). Growing up near or being in nature benefits children's social-emotional development. More so, research shows that these children may demonstrate higher rates of pro-environmental behaviors (Dopko et al., 2019), an added and significant benefit. Because children are spending less time outside than previous generations, opportunities to enhance positive social-emotional and pro-environmental behaviors through nature contact must become a priority. Outdoor learning that embraces hands-on exploration offers emotional experiences not found inside. Play does, as well.

The intrinsic and extrinsic value of play—which is the core of this book—cannot be trivialized or devalued. Children learn through play (Blalock et al., 2019). Play is also recognized as a protective factor, buffering the impact of at-risk or poor childhoods on mental and physical health (Whitebread, 2017). Outdoor play enhances this buffering effect (Quibell et al., 2017). Interestingly, the inherent danger level associated with risky play (explored in Chapter 3, "History and Value of Outdoor Play") can enhance a child's self-confidence, resilience, and social skills, not

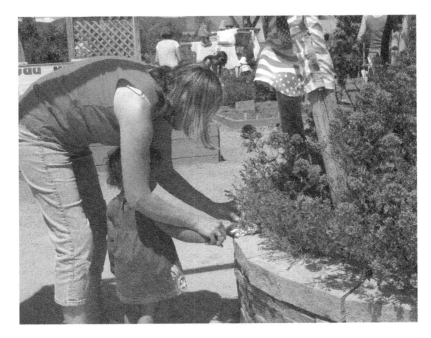

FIGURE 4.3   A shared moment with nature. Credit- author.

to mention physical health and well-being (Brussoni et al., 2015). Depending on how they are designed, play spaces in public parks or on school properties provide children with opportunities to be outside, play, enhance social-emotional skills, and increase physical activity (Raney et al., 2019) (see Figure 4.3).

The take-home message is that, for the sake of children's social-emotional development, ensure they *play*, *play* outside, and *play* outside often. Do not overlook the potential of including opportunities for risky play (as tolerated by your client) in an outdoor play space. Please see Table 4.2 for a comprehensive chart of social-emotional developmental milestones.

Cognitive Development

Cognition refers to the many components associated with thinking. *Cognitive development* is the broad process and sequence of acquiring knowledge and understanding (Davis et al., 2011; Paquin et al., 2020). Cognitive skills include reasoning, judgment, categorizing, memory, cause-and-effect, attention, decision-making, and problem-solving (Cherry, 2022; Mangin et al., 2017). During childhood, children enhance their cognitive repertoire through active engagement with the social and physical environment (Yildirim & Özyılmaz Akamca, 2017). Like social-emotional development, quality interaction with caregivers influences cognition. In schools and childcare centers, physical qualities such as lighting conditions, air quality, sound, and the condition and age of the buildings where children learn affect learning (Li & Sullivan, 2016).

Higher level skills, often referred to as *executive functions*, such as judgment, decision-making, and problem-solving, are guided by the prefrontal cortex, the most "forward" part of the brain (closest to the forehead). Because the prefrontal cortex is not fully developed until a person reaches their mid-20s, cognitive development is not completed until early adulthood. This lag in development can lead to poor decision-making and risky behaviors, particularly in adolescents. Please see Table 4.2 for a comprehensive chart of cognitive and language developmental milestones.

A major part of cognitive development is language, sometimes considered a developmental process of its own. If you have children or have had the opportunity to observe language development, you have seen that the process is amazing. To go from random sounds to the first meaningful words in a year is incredible. In fact, part of language development is reciprocal communication—dialogue. Long before infants say their first meaningful word, this process unfolds. One of the most important milestones of infancy is beginning to share attention with others (Cameron-Faulkner et al., 2021) as a bridge to communicating. Repeating back the sounds babies make is an early form of dialogue, especially when the baby "continues" the conversation. Box 4.2 outlines the typical stages of language acquisition.

BOX 4.2   EARLY LANGUAGE DEVELOPMENT SEQUENCE

Makes random sounds
Coos
Forms consonant sounds (e.g., t, b, m, n)
Babbles
Imitates consonant vowel patterns
Says first word(s)

Play, Nature, and Cognitive Development

The importance and value of outdoor play and its impact on learning cannot be underestimated. Extensive research shows that being outside matters—in a good way. Outdoor play that contains elements of exploration and discovery enhances learning and curiosity (Bento & Dias, 2017). Greener schoolyards and nearby nature are associated with higher academic test scores and overall academic achievement, even when controlling for socioeconomic status (Kuo et al., 2018; Li & Sullivan,

2016). Sustained attention is a key to learning, and contact with nature provides many such affordances for learning (Li & Sullivan, 2016). Being outside is a "natural" laboratory to learn and better understand new words and concepts such as observation, measurement, decision-making, and cause-and-effect (Yildirim & Özyılmaz Akamca, 2017).

Contrary to conventional views that nature distracts, preliminary research findings show that children are more engaged in classroom work right after learning outside. In addition—given that children are not getting enough exercise—walking from the classroom to an outdoor learning area and back provides physical activity, another cognitive boost (Kuo et al., 2018). Over the long term, learning that occurs outside speeds up the acquisition and retrieval of new knowledge.

Connectedness of Development

What follows is a short, fictitious case study about outdoor play. It demonstrates how complex and interconnected development is with social and physical environmental contexts (*specified in parentheses*) and how each development area depends on the others to "build a whole child."

> Six-year-olds Luca and Caleb, best friends for the past 3 years (*social-emotional context*), are playing together (*social-emotional* and *emotional*) on the blacktop at their urban elementary school (*physical*). It is a special day: The supervising teacher has brought out a large bin full of hoops, balls, baskets, and ribbons (*gross and fine motor*) for the children to play with on the blacktop because space is limited elsewhere on the school grounds (*physical*). The only other outdoor space is a small climbing structure and a freestanding metal slide (*gross motor* and *physical*). Luca and Caleb grasp hands (*social-emotional* and *emotional*) and run (*gross motor*) to the bin.
>
> So do many other children, all of them excited by the novelty of new playthings. They want access to these special items (*social-emotional* and *emotional*). There is a bit of a skirmish at the bin; children engage in name-calling (*social-emotional*) and jostling (*gross motor*) with each other to get the best access (*social-emotional*).
>
> Quickly recognizing a situation that could easily go awry (*cognitive* and *emotional*), the teacher says in a loud but gentle voice, "Little chickadees, flap your wings five times (*cognitive* and *gross motor*) and fly to your nest (*gross motor*)." She gestures with her arms (wings!) to the area around the bin (*cognitive* and *social-emotional*).
>
> Captivated, the children scramble to find an open space so that they can land in their metaphoric nests (*cognitive, gross motor,* and *physical*). Luca and Caleb flap their wings five times, counting aloud (*cognitive* and *gross motor*), and fly to their nest. There, Luca kneels, and Caleb sits cross-legged (*gross motor*), both eagerly listening for the teacher's next directions (*cognitive*).

The teacher explains that are enough bins, baskets, and the like for everyone. She instructs the children to ever-so-quietly tap their fingers and thumbs together like hungry birds opening and closing their beaks (*cognitive* and *fine motor*), stand up, stretch their wings—and when she calls their names—fly to the bin and pick two objects (*cognitive, gross* and *fine motor*).

After all the children receive their two objects and find a place to create, play begins. Many children share their treasures to construct all types of creative products (*cognitive, gross* and *fine motor, social-emotional,* and *social*). Chatter and laughter abound (*cognitive, social-emotional,* and *social*). Noting no conflicts that require her intervention, the teacher remains in the background and watches the play unfold (*cognitive* and *social-emotional*). Unsurprisingly, the theme spontaneously becomes bird-focused: Nests are woven from the ribbons, baskets are filled with imaginary feed, and hoops become nest frames (*cognitive* and *fine motor*). What a great day at school it is!

To further illustrate the interconnectedness of development, Table 4.2 provides a detailed timeline and list of developmental norms from birth through adolescence (0–18 years) (see Figure 4.4).

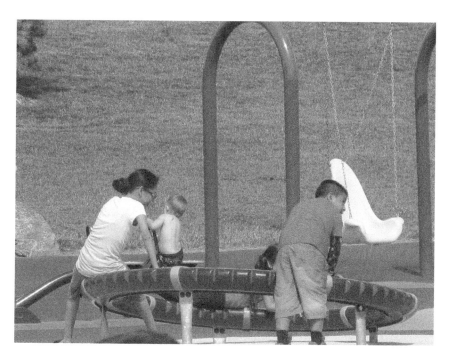

FIGURE 4.4   One play element can simultaneously support motor, social-emotional, and cognitive development. Credit- author.

Final Thoughts

In this chapter, we presented an overview of childhood development intended to guide design decision-making. There is nothing simple about development; everything about it is interconnected, and nothing happens in isolation. For most children, the process proceeds as expected. This is not the case for other children, who rely on physical and emotional environmental modifications—that designers and planners need to be part of—so they can participate in life and engage in childhood activities that are fun, meaningful, and support their future development.

BOX 4.3   CASE STUDY: THE AWESOME SPOT PLAYGROUND (FIGURES 4.5–4.7)

Project Information:

Name
The Awesome Spot Playground

Designer
O'Dell Engineering

Location
Modesto, CA

Size
6,400 m² or 1.58 acres

Year Built
2022

Age Group(s)
2–5 years, 5–12 years, intergenerational

Description:

This play space is a heartfelt, impassioned project centered around one local family's desire for their son, Tommy, to be able to play freely. Tommy Loredo was born with severe physical abnormalities and congenital deformities that would require many years of intense therapy, surgeries, and uncertainty. The space brings together evidence-based sensory integration research, technologically advanced, socially inclusive, and physically accessible play in the heart of California's Central Valley.

This play space exceeds standard "accessible" play. In addition to exceeding ADA standards, the Awesome Spot serves as an opportunity for community members of all ages, abilities (physical, sensory, or cognitive), genders, and sociocultural and sociogeographical backgrounds to play and interact easily and effectively. Based on community input, play is divided into three distinct areas for exploration and free play: the Swamp Cruise, the Savannah Safari, and the Rainforest Excursion. Each area contains a multitude of sensory-rich experiences offering graduated difficulty levels, "just right" sensory input, and exploratory play opportunities. Site planning for the project was purposeful to promote play through cognitive simplicity, social interaction, and multisensory experiences without the use of ramps. All walkways are designed with less than 5% slopes to significantly limit the physical effort needed to access high points in the play spaces.

Website:

- http://www.theawesomespotplayground.com/

Traditional Inclusive Features	Inclusive+ Features
• Accessible path of travel • Accessible structures • Accessible swings • PIP rubber surfacing • Accessible slides • Accessible climbers • Completely fenced perimeter for safety	• Having no ramps limits the required physical effort to navigate the play space • Nature-based theme to enhance exploratory play options • Double-wide roller slide to encourage social play • Multiple cozy spaces for self-regulation and restoration • Multisystem sensory walls to experience all the sensory systems • Roll-under capacity in raised water play that encourages social interaction and sensory play • Self-cleaning, inclusive restroom with adult-size changing table and lift • Integrated landscape and natural elements to encourage loose-parts play • Integrated grade changes that provide movement challenges • Overarching play approach focused on social integration • Intergenerational play options to bring families and caregivers together • Companion seating benches and tables for comfort and socialization • Themed zones and path hierarchy for ease of understanding • 18 accessible parking stalls maximize access to the play space • Integrated and natural shade options to help with temperature regulation • Designed with and built as a unified community

Remarks:

This play space is the culmination of a multiyear endeavor of combined efforts from city and county governments, school districts, local service groups, philanthropic corporations, and grassroots community advocates. The team effort—from creating the original design to completing construction—was truly a unifying experience for the community. The inclusive⁺ nature of this space transcends basic accessibility to embrace the individual differences that make the community stronger and more vibrant. The concept is that all patrons should be able to enjoy each and every aspect of the site. The concept is embodied in the fact that all areas, whether high or low, are infused with interesting and playful activities that place the user in a creative and dramatic world where individual differences enhance the experience. An example custom play feature is the aviary perch, which transforms the user into an imaginary singing bird soaring 10 feet above play activities—while across the play space, children can play among safari animals roaming across the savannah. These are just two of many inclusive⁺ play features that foster social interaction, sensory immersion, creativity, and intergenerational interaction for everyone.

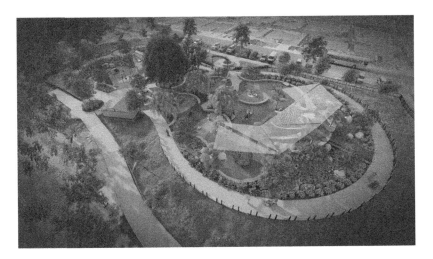

FIGURE 4.5 Bird's eye view. Credit- author.

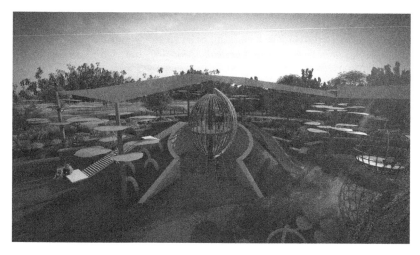

FIGURE 4.6   The Rain Forest Excursion area features an inclusive[+] area with graded challenges and the most interesting feature at the highest possible location. Credit- author.

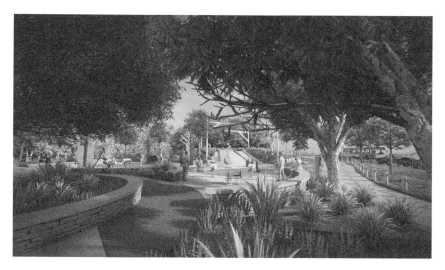

FIGURE 4.7   The Savanna Safari area offers active and passive movement and sensorial activities. Credit- author.

References

Bento, G., & Dias, G. (2017). The importance of outdoor play for young children's healthy development. *Porto Biomedical Journal, 2*(5), 157–160. https://doi.org/10.1016/j.pbj.2017.03.003

Berk, L. (2018a). *Exploring child and adolescent development.* Pearson.

Berk, L. (2018b). *Exploring child development.* Pearson.

Berger, K. S. (2019). *The developing person through the life span* (11th ed.). Worth.

Bornstein, M. H., Britto, P. R., Nonoyama-Tarumi, Y., Ota, Y., Petrovic, O., & Putnick, D. L. (2012). Child development in developing countries: Introduction and methods. *Child Development, 83*(1), 16–31. https://doi.org/10.1111/j.1467-8624.2011.01671.x

Bowlby, J. (1988). *A secure base.* Basic Books.

Blalock, S. M., Lindo, N., & Ray, D. C. (2019). Individual and group child-centered play therapy: Impact on social-emotional competencies. *Journal of Counseling & Development, 97*(3), 238–249. https://doi.org/10.1002/jcad.12264

Bronfenbrenner, U. (1979). *Ecology of human development.* Harvard University Press.

Bronfenbrenner, U. (1986). Ecology of the family as a context for human development: Research perspectives. Developmental Psychology, 22(6), 723–742.

Bronfenbrenner, U., & Morris, P. A. (1998). The ecology of developmental processes. In W. Damon & R. M. Lerner (Eds.), *Handbook of child psychology: Vol. 1. Theoretical models of human development* (5th ed., pp. 993–1028). John Wiley & Sons.

Brussoni, M., Gibbons, R., Gray, C., Ishikawa, T., Sandseter, E. B. H., Bienenstock, A., Chabot, G., Fuselli, P., Herrington, S., Janssen, I., Pickett, W., Power, M., Stanger, N., Sampson, M., & Tremblay, M. S. (2015). What is the relationship between risky outdoor play and health in children? A systematic review. *International Journal of Environmental Research and Public Health, 12*(6), 6423–6454. https://doi.org/10.3390/ijerph120606423

Cameron-Faulkner, T., Malik, N., Steele, C., Coretta, S., Serratrice, L., & Lieven, E. (2021). A cross-cultural analysis of early prelinguistic gesture development and its relationship to language development. *Child Development, 92*(1), 273–290. https://doi.org/10.1111/cdev.13406

Cherry, K. (2022). *What is cognition?* Very Well Mind. https://www.verywellmind.com/what-is-cognition-2794982

Craig, G. J., & Baucum, D. (2002). *Human development* (9th ed.). Pearson.

Davies, D. (1999). *Child development: A practitioner's guide.* Guilford Press.

Davis, E. E., Pitchford, N. J., & Limback, E. (2011). The interrelation between cognitive and motor development in typically developing children aged 4–11 years is under-pinned by visual processing and fine manual control. *British Journal of Psychology, 102*(3), 569–584. https://doi.org/10.1111/j.2044-8295.2011.02018.x

Denham, S. A., Wyatt, T. M., Bassett, H. H., Echeverria, D., & Knox, S. S. (2009). Assessing social-emotional development in children from a longitudinal perspective. *Journal of Epidemiology & Community Health, 63*(Suppl 1), i37–i52. https://doi.org/10.1136/jech.2007.070797

Dettweiler, U., Becker, C., Auestad, B. H., Simon, P., & Kirsch, P. (2017). Stress in school. Some empirical hints on the circadian cortisol rhythm of children in outdoor and indoor classes. *International Journal of Environmental Research and Public Health, 14*(5), 475. https://doi.org/10.3390/ijerph14050475

Dopko, R. L., Capaldi, C. A., & Zelenski, J. M. (2019). The psychological and social benefits of a nature experience for children: A preliminary investigation. *Journal of Environmental Psychology, 63*, 134–138. https://doi.org/10.1016/j.jenvp.2019.05.002

Dunn, W. L., & Craig, G. L. (2006). *Understanding human development.* Prentice Hall.

Durlak, J. A., Weissberg, R. P., Dymnicki, A. B., Taylor, R. D., & Schellinger, K. B. (2011). The impact of enhancing students' social and emotional learning: A meta-analysis of school-based universal interventions. *Child Development, 82*(1), 405–432. https://doi.org/10.1111/j.1467-8624.2010.01564.x

Emde, R. N., Gaensbauer, T. J., & Harmon, R. J. (1976). *Emotional expression in infancy.* International Universities Press.

Erhardt, R. (1982). *Developmental Prehension Assessment.* Ramsco.

Erikson, E. (1963). Childhood and society. W. W. Norton.

Erikson, E. (1982). The life cycle completed. W. W. Norton.

Feldman, R. S. (2016). *Development across the lifespan* (8th ed.). Prentice Hall.

Folger, A. T., Putnam, K. T., Putnam, F. W., Peugh, J. L., Eismann, E. A., Sa, T., Shapiro, R. A., Van Ginkel, J. B., & Ammerman, R. T. (2017). Maternal interpersonal trauma and child social-emotional development: An intergenerational effect. *Paediatric and Perinatal Epidemiology, 31*(2), 99–107. https://doi.org/10.1111/ppe.12341

Harvard Center on the Developing Child. (2020). *Connecting the brain to the rest of the body.* Harvard University. https://46y5eh11fhgw3ve3ytpwxt9r-wpengine.netdna-ssl.com/wp-content/uploads/2020/06/InBrief-Connecting-the-Brain-to-the-Rest-of-the-Body.pdf

Jacobs, K., & Jacobs, L. (2014). *Quick reference dictionary for occupational therapy* (6th ed.). SLACK.

Kagan, J. (1984). *The nature of the child.* Basic Books.

Kit, B. K., Akinbami, L. J., Isfahani, N. S., & Ulrich, D. A. (2017). Gross motor development in children aged 3–5 Years, United States 2012. *Maternal and Child Health Journal, 21*(7), 1573–1580. https://doi.org/10.1007/s10995-017-2289-9

Kuo, M., Browning, M. H. E. M., & Penner, M. L. (2018). Do lessons in nature boost subsequent classroom engagement? Refueling students in flight. *Frontiers in Psychology, 8*, Article 2253. https://doi.org/10.3389/fpsyg.2017.02253

Laaksoharju, T., Rappe, E., & Kaivola, T. (2012). Garden affordances for social learning, plat, and for building nature-child relationship. *Urban Forestry & Urban Greening, 11*(2), 195–203. https://doi.org/10.1016/j.ufug.2012.01.003

Li, D., & Sullivan, W. C. (2016). Impact of views to school landscapes on recovery from stress and mental fatigue. *Landscape and Urban Planning, 148*, 149–158. https://doi.org/10.1016/j.landurbplan.2015.12.015

Logigan, M. K., & Ward, J. D. (1989). *Pediatric rehabilitation.* Little, Brown.

Mangin, K. S., Horwood, L. J., & Woodward, L. J. (2017). Cognitive development trajectories of very preterm and typically developing children. *Child Development, 88*(1), 282–298. https://doi.org/10.1111/cdev.12585

Maslow, A. (1968). Toward a psychology of being (2nd ed.). Van Nostrand Reinhold.

Maslow, A. (1970). Motivation and personality (2nd ed.). Harper and Row.

Paquin, C., Côté, S. M., Tremblay, R. E., Séguin, J. R., Boivin, M., & Herba, C. M. (2020). Maternal depressive symptoms and children's cognitive development: Does early childcare and child's sex matter? *PLoS ONE, 15*(1), Article e0227179. https://doi.org/10.1371/journal.pone.0227179

Piaget, J., & Inhelder, B. (1969). *The psychology of the child* (6th ed.). Prentice Hall.

Quibell, T., Charlton, J., & Law, J. (2017). Wilderness schooling: A controlled trial of the impact of an outdoor education programme on attainment outcomes in primary school pupils. *British Educational Research Journal, 43*(3), 572–587. https://doi.org/10.1002/berj.3273

Raney, M. A., Hendry, C. F., & Yee, S. A. (2019). Physical activity and social behaviors of urban children in green playgrounds. *American Journal of Preventive Medicine, 56*(4), 522–529. https://doi.org/10.1016/j.amepre.2018.11.004

Rapee, R. M., Oar, E. L., Johnco, C. J., Forbes, M. K., Fardouly, J., Natasha, R., Magson, N. R., & Richardson, C. E. (2019). Adolescent development and risk for the onset of social-emotional disorders: A review and conceptual model. *Behavior Research and Therapy, 123*, Article 103501. https://doi.org/10.1016/j.brat.2019.103501

Santrock, J. W. (2018). *Children* (17th ed.). McGraw Hill.

Shaffer, D. R. (2013). *Developmental psychology: Childhood and adolescence* (9th ed.). Wadsworth.

Shonkoff, J. P., & Phillips, D. A. (2000). *From neurons to neighborhoods: The science of early childhood development.* National Academy Press.

Steinberg, L., Bornstein, M. H., Vandell, D. L., & Rook, K. S. (2010). *Lifespan development: Infancy through adulthood.* Cengage Learning.

Stern, D. (1985). *The interpersonal world of the child.* Basic Books.

Treat, A. E., Sheffield-Morris, A., Williamson, A. C., & Hays-Grudo, J. (2020). Adverse childhood experiences and young children's social and emotional development: The role of maternal depression, self-efficacy, and social support. *Early Child Development and Care, 190*(15), 2422–2436. https://doi.org/10.1080/03004430.2019.1578220

Velikonjia, T., Edbrooke-Childs, J., Calderon, A., Sleed, M., Brown, A., & Deighton, J. (2017). The psychometric properties of the Ages & Stages Questionnaires for ages 2–2.5: A systematic review. *Child: Care, Health, and Development, 43*(1), 1–17. https://doi.org/10.1111/cch.12397

VORT Corporation. (2010). *Hawaii early learning profile: 3–6 years* (2nd ed.). VORT. https://www.vort.com/home.php?cat=2

Vygotsky, L. (1978). *Mind in society.* Harvard University Press.

Wagenfeld, A. (2017). A snapshot of early development. In A. Wagenfeld, J. Kaldenberg, & D. Honaker (Eds.), *Foundations of pediatric practice for the occupational therapy assistant* (2nd ed., pp. 59–68). SLACK, Inc.

Wagenfeld, A., Kaldenberg, J., & Honaker, D. (2017). *Foundations of pediatric practice for the occupational therapy assistant* (2nd ed.). SLACK, Inc.

Walker, S. P., Wachs, T. D., Grantham-McGregor, S., Black, M. M., Nelson, C. A., Huffman, S. L., Baker-Henningham, H., Chang, S. M., Hamadani, J. D., Lozoff, B., Gardner, J. M. M., Powell, C. A., Rahman, A., & Richter, L. (2011). Inequality in early childhood: Risk and protective factors for early child development. *The Lancet, 378*(9799), 1325–1338. https://doi.org/10.1016/S0140-6736(11)60555-2

Wells, N. M., & Evans, G. W. (2003). Nearby nature: A buffer of life stress among rural children. *Environment and Behavior, 35*(3), 311–330. https://doi.org/10.1177/0013916503035003001

Whitebread, D. (2017). Free play and children's mental health. *The Lancet Child & Adolescent Health, 1*(3), 167–169. https://doi.org/10.1016/S2352-4642(17)30092-5

World Health Organization. (2007). *International classification of functioning, disability and health: Children & youth version; ICF-CY.* https://apps.who.int/iris/bitstream/handle/10665/43737/9789241547321_eng.pdf

Yidirim, G., & Özyılmaz Akamca, G. (2017). The effect of outdoor learning activities on the development of preschool children. *South African Journal of Education, 37*(2), 1–10. https://doi.org/10.15700/saje.v37n2a1378

5

SENSORY INTEGRATION

Why It Matters

What are you doing right now? Of course, you are reading this chapter, which means you are looking or listening—but what else? Are you sitting or lying down? How does the surface feel? Does it have a smell? If your chair has wheels or can rock, are you making use of either? Are you having a snack or a meal while you read? If yes, is your drink hot or cold? Is the food salty, sweet, crunchy, or smooth? So many more things than reading or listening to the chapter are happening with your sensory systems, and each one plays an important role in helping you stay focused and organized.

Introduction

Every day and in each moment of our lives, we take in, screen, sort, and manage sensory information from the environment. Our daily lives are shaped by multi-sensory experiences. We use the constant flow of information to help organize our emotions and behaviors, learn, and interact with the world. This amazing process is called *sensory integration,* a neurological process that involves taking in and responding to sensory information. The process works well for most people with little thought about it. It enables us to play, work, socialize, and care for ourselves. Sensory integration is important.

You are likely familiar with the five basic senses: vision, hearing, taste, smell, and touch. However, there are three other foundational sensory systems to consider: proprioceptive, vestibular, and interoceptive. All eight sensory systems need to integrate and work together because they play a crucial role in helping us function in our daily lives and regulate our thoughts and actions. All eight of our sensory systems do what they need to do for most people. We do not have to think about what each sense is contributing to an activity; it just happens. Chalk drawing

DOI: 10.4324/9781003193890-5

is one example from outdoor play that uses all the sensory systems except taste. When we explore the eight sensory systems later in this chapter, we share how this simple activity—chalk drawing—is, perhaps, more complex than you imagine because it is so multisensory.

Life can be very challenging and overwhelming for children and adults whose sensory systems are not organized, integrated, or working in sync. About 5% of all kindergarten-age children experience sensory integrative difficulties. For children with autism spectrum disorder, the prevalence of sensory integrative challenges ranges from 40% to 90% (Ben-Sasson et al., 2009; Pfeiffer et al., 2018). Please note that many people have sensory "quirks." They may shun fabric textures that feel itchy or uncomfortable, avoid swings because they make them dizzy, or dislike certain smells. Those reactions are on the spectrum of normal. Instead, what we are talking about in this chapter are children whose sensory systems are so dysregulated that daily activities are difficult to initiate, do, and complete. Their social relationships are difficult to develop and maintain because of the sensory integration challenges they experience. Life is hard.

This chapter is not intended to instruct the application of sensory integration theory; trained occupational therapists most frequently provide that highly specialized therapeutic intervention. Nevertheless, there are good reasons to have a basic understanding of sensory integration as part of excellent design practice. We use this chapter to provide that foundation. We explore the eight sensory systems, introduce sensory integration, and delve into why it is vital to consider sensory integration and sensation when designing inclusive[+] outdoor play spaces.

Sensation

The Merriam-Webster (n.d.) online dictionary defines *sensation* as "a mental process (such as seeing, hearing, or smelling) resulting from the immediate external stimulation of a sense organ." We perceive sensation from the environment, process it in the central nervous system (the brain and spinal cord), and then respond with some action. As we shared earlier, the basic premise of sensory integration—perceive, process, and respond—is a well-oiled feedback loop continually operating in the background, doing what it needs to do without us paying much attention. For most people, that feedback loop does its job. Let's use the auditory system as an example:

> *I (Amy) am sitting outside on my balcony right now, writing this chapter. A large office building is being built across the street, and I have gotten used to the day-to-day construction noises. However, just a few minutes ago, a loud bang made me jump.*

The loop was: (1) perceive: an unexpected noise (external stimulation), (2) process: my brain registered this noise as unfamiliar, and (3) respond: my response was to jump (action). It happened quickly, and before I knew it, I recovered from my initial startle and was back at work, writing unbothered with no lingering aftereffects. This is not the case for children (and adults) with sensory integrative challenges.

What Is a Sensory System?

A sensory system contains sensory receptors, neural pathways, and brain structures. Humans have eight sensory systems. As we shared in the Introduction, five sensory systems are typically referred to as the basic senses: auditory, gustatory, olfactory, tactile, and visual. The remaining three sensory systems—proprioceptive, vestibular, and interoceptive—are the foundational sensory systems, meaning they are the first to develop in utero (see Figure 5.1).

Although all eight sensory systems are important in daily life, the focus of sensory integration therapy is the foundational proprioceptive, vestibular, and interoceptive systems and, to a lesser extent, the tactile, auditory, and visual systems. When the eight systems operate together and in sync, the entire sensory system is regulated, making it easier to manage and control emotions and behaviors. As discussed, most people's sensory systems are integrated. Because the physical environment substantially affects sensory integration and regulation, the sensory systems can over- or under-register or be spot-on—and designers can contribute to sensory regulation. We have found that the best, most effective, and client-centered way to create effective sensory spaces (indoor and outdoor) is through interdisciplinary collaboration between landscape architects and occupational therapists.

All Eight Sensory Systems

With that brief introduction, let's explore all eight sensory systems. We begin with the five basic senses and then move to the three foundational sensory systems.

Auditory System (Hearing)

The auditory system enables us to hear. Being able to hear is protective and plays a significant role in communication. *We are not saying that individuals who are deaf or hard of hearing cannot communicate; that is not at all the case. We are discussing the auditory system's function and purpose.* The auditory system has two parts, the peripheral system (called such because it is outside the central nervous system) and the central system. The peripheral system contains the outer, middle, and inner ear and the auditory nerve, which carries information from the cochlea in the inner ear to the brain. The central system contains auditory pathways in the brain stem and auditory cortex part of the brain (Lobe, n.d.). More than being responsible for sending sound information, the auditory system also provides cues about the sound's frequency, volume, and location in space (where it is coming from; Lobe, n.d.) (see Figure 5.2).

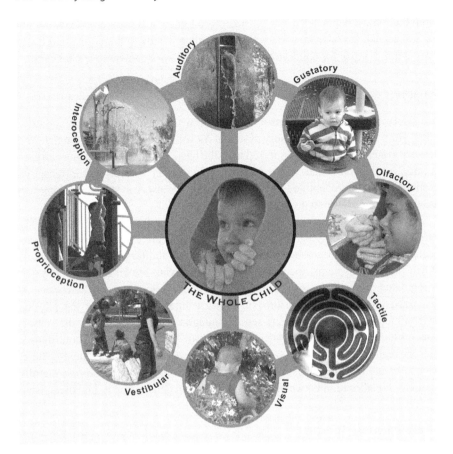

FIGURE 5.1 The eight sensory systems. Credit- author.

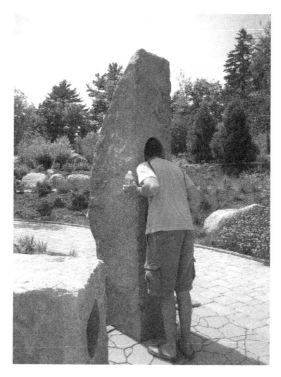

FIGURE 5.2   Multi height naturalized sound chambers for seated and standing users. Credit- author.

Visual System (Seeing)

We perceive the world around us through light. Vision and visual perception are the processes of receiving information from the environment as light and then analyzing, interpreting, and making sense of that information (Price & Remington, 2012). Vision begins with the eye. Images are formed through a process called *refraction*, a bending of light rays that travel from one transparent medium to another (National Eye Institute, 2022). The visual system is highly complex. Each component serves a specific function that coordinates and contributes to both seeing and understanding what is seen. The components are the eye, optic nerve, optic chiasm, optic tract, lateral geniculate nucleus, optic radiation, visual cortex, and visual association cortex (Sincero, 2013). It is beyond the scope of this chapter to detail each visual system component; however, we provide a basic overview of the anatomy of the eye.

Eyelids. Eyelids cover and protect the anterior (front) surface of the eye. They
    contain glands that make lubricating tear film.
Sclera. The sclera is the white portion of the eyeball. It is an opaque white color
    because it is composed of collagen fibers. The muscles that enable the eyeball to
    move are located in the sclera.

Lens. The lens is considered the eye's "accommodator." It changes shape when the eye focuses on an object, flattening when the eye focuses on something in the distance and thickening when the eye looks at something close.

Cornea. The cornea is the structure of the eye where light waves enter. The cornea and the lens work together to bend (refract) the light waves onto the retina.

Extraocular muscles. These muscles move the eye and its orbit.

Iris. The iris holds the eye's pigmentation or color.

Pupil. The pupil is located in the center of the iris, where light enters. Reflexively, the pupil expands or dilates in low light and narrows or constricts in bright light. After refracting in the cornea and lens, the light rays travel to the pupil en route to the retina.

Retina. The retina, located at the back of the eye, contains neural tissue. Light energy is converted to signals through a complex biochemical process in the neural tissues. The signals travel along a neural pathway, passing through the retina to the optic nerve. From there, the signals are routed to other places in the brain for visual (seeing) and visual perception (understanding what is seen) processing. The two types of photoreceptors located in the retina are rods and cones. *Rods* enable us to see in black, white, and grey; *cones* allow us to see in color. What we see happens in the retina.

Optic nerve. The optic nerve, located at the back of the brain, is responsible for carrying visual information from the visual system to the brain.

Optic chiasm. The point where the optic nerve from one eye meets and crosses the optic nerve from the other eye is termed the optic chiasm. Here, information from both eyes is joined. The optic chiasm is located at the base of the hypothalamus in the brain (Price & Remington, 2012, p. 1; Sincero, 2013).

Olfactory System (Smell)

The olfactory system enables us to smell. Although the human sense of smell is not as acute as, for example, a dog's, we can detect one trillion smells, which is no small feat (Bushdid et al., 2014). Smell is a highly protective sense; the odor of smoke evokes awareness of danger and a fight-or-flight response. Smell and taste are closely related; for many people, the smell and taste of freshly baked cookies are tantalizing. The sense of smell begins at the back of the nose with a strip of neurons called the *olfactory epithelium* (Curley, 2015). Once the sensory receptors are activated in the olfactory epithelium, an electrical signal is sent to the *olfactory bulb* at the base of the forebrain and then to other areas in the brain to identify the smell. Unlike the other sensory systems, odors are processed first in the emotion and memory area of the brain, the limbic system, before traveling to the thalamus. The smell–taste connection occurs in the thalamus, a relay station for all sensory information from the eight senses coming into the brain. The thalamus sends the smell information to the orbitofrontal cortex, where it integrates with taste information (Curley, 2015). What we consider taste is actually the integration of smell and taste.

Gustatory System (Taste)

The gustatory system is located in the mouth and tongue, which have specialized cells that send messages to the brain to decode five specific tastes. These five taste sensations are sweet, sour, salty, bitter, and umami. The bitter sensation is protective; sometimes, bitter is equated with poisonous. *Umami,* frequently mentioned in the "foodie world," is a savory or delicious taste. There are taste cells in the taste buds, which are visible if you look at your tongue. They look like little raised bumps.

Another component of the gustatory system is the common chemical sense (SPD Australia, n.d.a). It comprises many nerve endings in the eyes, nose, mouth, and throat. These nerve endings are responsible for sensations, such as the sting we feel when cutting onions and the irritation we experience from hot peppers. Combined, the five taste sensations, the common chemical sense, food texture, temperature, and odor produce a perception of flavor. Now that you know taste and smell are tightly linked, try this experiment: Hold your nose while eating a piece of chocolate. Although you will likely identify whether it is sweet or bitter, can you taste the "chocolate-ness"?

Tactile System (Touch)

The tactile system is responsible for interpreting touch, pressure, vibration, temperature, and pain information through the skin. It then sends the information via tactile nerve receptors and pathways to the *somatosensory cortex* (brainstem, spinal cord, and thalamus) for processing (Star Institute, n.d.). Touch receptors are located everywhere on the body but mainly on the skin. They provide information about the dimensions, shapes, and textures of objects. Because the skin covers the entire body, the tactile system is the largest sensory system.

Can you think of anything we do that does not involve touch? In some capacity, we experience tactile input every moment of our lives: Whether we are sitting, lying down, running, jumping, walking, working at the computer, bathing, or eating, at least one part of our body is always in contact with something in the environment.

There are two layers of skin; the outermost is the *epidermis*, and the thick layer beneath it is the *dermis*. The touch (tactile) receptors are located at nerve endings in this thick layer, the dermis. Six kinds of tactile receptors in the skin allow us to experience touch (Raising an Extraordinary Person, n.d.):

Meissner's corpuscles. Meissner's corpuscles are sensory receptors nearest the skin's surface and perceive fine touch, pressure, and vibration. When Meissner's corpuscles are deformed by pressure, they send neural signals to the brain.

Merkel's disks. Merkel's disks are receptive to light touch.

Ruffini endings. Ruffini endings detect when the skin is being stretched and perceive temperature and pressure.

Pacinian corpuscles. Pacinian corpuscles detect deep-pressure sensations.

Krause's end bulbs. Krause's end bulbs are sensitive to cold.

Free nerve endings. Free nerve endings are generic receptors that respond to pressure, temperature, pain, and texture.

Vestibular System (Balance)

The vestibular system, one of the foundational sensory systems, comprises mainly the structures in the middle ear. This system provides the brain with information about movement, the position of the head, and the body's position in space. It is the major player in the movement patterns that keep us upright and balanced, and it helps maintain our bodies in a stable position. You might think of the vestibular system as the "dizzy" system. Vestibular experiences include boating, swinging, spinning, rolling, and rocking—which some people find regulating and calming, but others find extremely unpleasant. As we age, our tolerance for vestibular input declines. Carnival rides no longer hold much or any appeal, and riding in the backseat of a car can be nauseating. An intact vestibular system enables us to maintain normal movement and equilibrium.

Receptors in the middle ear send messages to the brain, specifically to the cerebellum, which is the part of the brain responsible for coordinating muscular activity for processing and response. There is a strong connection between the vestibular

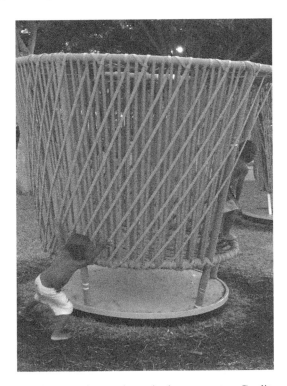

FIGURE 5.3   The Los Trompos innovative spinning apparatus. Credit- author.

and visual systems, as well as between the vestibular and proprioceptive systems. Think about it: When you are dizzy, can you see straight or maintain an upright posture? Can you understand where your body is in space; what is up and what is down? (see Figure 5.3).

Proprioceptive System (Body Position in Space and Movement)

Another foundational sensory system, the proprioceptive system, controls movement and posture. *Proprioception* is the sensation of joint movement and acceleration. This sensory system helps us understand where our bodies are in space. Many people find proprioceptive input to be very calming. We receive proprioceptive input from activities like carrying and pushing heavy loads, jumping, squeezing into tight spaces, doing pushups, hanging from monkey bars, and wearing a lead apron at the dentist's office. All these activities involve muscle and joint activation.

Proprioceptors, such as muscle spindles, monitor muscle length, tension, and pressure. Fine motor activities (small hand movements, such as stringing beads, drawing, or deadheading flowers) require a greater density of muscle spindles than do gross motor activities (large movements, such as running or throwing a ball). Muscle spindles are very important because the brain needs information from them to register changes in the muscles' angles and positions. The arms and legs are instrumental in maintaining posture against gravity (activities such as standing up), so many muscle spindles are located in the arms and legs.

Another proprioceptor is the Golgi tendon organs, which are found wherever muscle meets tendon in the body. These organs send information about tension in specific muscle parts to the brain. There are also proprioceptors in the joints and ligaments that, again, are responsible for sending information about the movement to the brain. Proprioceptors can also be found in the middle ear, which, along with the vestibular system, helps regulate motion, balance, and the body's orientation in space. As with the other sensory systems, information coming into the central nervous system is processed and sent back. In the case of the proprioceptive system, information is sent to the muscles and joints for a response (or movement). Sometimes, depending on multiple factors, this movement is done consciously or automatically (SPD Australia, n.d.b.) (see Figure 5.4).

Interoceptive System (Internal Regulation)

The interoceptive system, an important foundational sensory system often overlooked in indoor and outdoor space design, is the internal, "inside the body" sensory system. It has receptors on internal organs, bones, and the skin. Messages from these receptors are sent to your brain for processing and alert you, for example, that you are cold, hot, hungry, thirsty, need to use the restroom, or your heart is racing (see Figure 5.5).

There is a strong connection between interoception, emotions, and emotional experience. More broadly, there is a relationship between well-organized sensory

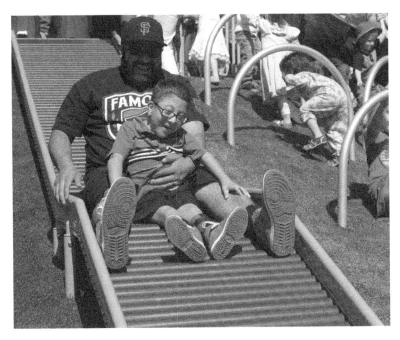

FIGURE 5.4   Shared joy on a sensory rich slide. Credit- Rachel Loredo.

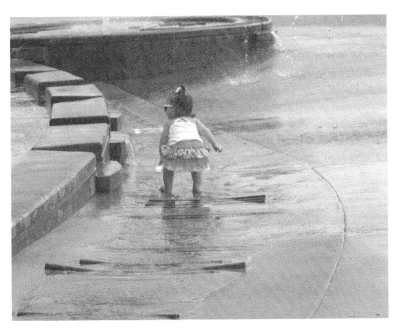

FIGURE 5.5   Water play is irresistibly fun and is a source of interoception. Credit- author.

systems and sound mental health. The limbic system is a set of brain regions associated with emotions and responsible, in part, for sensory registration (Kilroy et al., 2019). Lacking good awareness of interoceptive cues is associated with poor emotional regulation (Bennie, 2016; Price & Hooven, 2018). In fact, there is increasing interest within the health community in relationships between the sensory systems, particularly dysregulated or interrupted interoception, and trauma.

An awareness of interoceptive processes offers a window into regulating emotions, thinking, and body sensations (Craig, 2015; Khalsa & Lapidus, 2016). Imagine that you are about to enter an interview with a prospective client. Your heart is racing; your palms are sweaty; and, yes, you are nervous. Taking a slow four-count in and six-count out deep breath can help you reverse those interoceptive responses and regulate yourself. Here is another example: You are outside mowing the lawn. It is hot, and you are sweating. You start to feel frustrated that there is still a huge swath of unmown lawn that needs attention. Nothing sounds better than a huge glass of ice water. Again, your interoceptive sensory system is sending you a call-to-action message: Get that drink, sit under a tree, and rest for a bit.

The Chalk-Drawing Example

With this introduction to the eight sensory systems laid out, let's return to the chalk-drawing example from the Introduction. Chalk drawing is a versatile activity that many children and adults enjoy. It gets us moving and thinking and is sensory-rich, creative, and fun—and even more fun when done outside. Here is how to do a simple chalk-drawing activity (and the sensory systems it involves):

- Find a shady place to draw (visual, interoception)
- Open the container of chalk, select a color, and remove the piece of chalk from the container (auditory, visual, tactile, olfactory, proprioception)
- Grasp the chalk in your fingers or hand (visual, tactile, proprioception)
- Bring the hand holding the chalk to the writing surface, such as the sidewalk or paper (visual, tactile, vestibular, proprioception)
- Draw and repeat the process with other colors of chalk (auditory, visual, tactile, vestibular, proprioception)
- Return the chalk into the container (visual, tactile, olfactory, proprioception)
- Rinse down the sidewalk, as needed (auditory, visual, tactile, olfactory, vestibular, proprioception, interoception)

This simple example demonstrates that every task we do involves sensation and how important it is for the sensory systems to be regulated and integrated to participate successfully in life. Except for *taste* (we do not encourage eating chalk!), the remaining seven sensory systems are working hard in this example to make the activity flow and for children to feel capable and successful in creating chalk masterpieces.

Here is the flip side of chalk drawing: How might it feel if the smell of chalk was nauseating? If the sensation of the chalk contacting the sidewalk felt like needles throbbing through your arm? If the sound of chalk scratching on the sidewalk made you shiver with fear? If you could not shift your head and neck to adjust to drawing in different areas of the sidewalk or paper because it made you dizzy? If you had to use all your mental energy to think about staying on your knees or squatting to draw without falling? If you could not understand where your body is in space or how to use it most efficiently and, instead of pulling one piece of chalk at a time from the container, you pulled out three—and broke two putting them back—and the sun was beating down on you? That is a lot that can go awry, isn't it? A seemingly fun, simple, and desirable childhood activity would be anything but fun. Play needs to be fun. Although designers do not treat or "cure" sensory integration issues, they have an essential role in helping to create outdoor spaces that accommodate different sensory preferences and needs (see Figure 5.6).

Sensory Integration

Designers may not be familiar with sensory integration or the theory that explains it. *Sensory integration* is a theory and a specialized therapeutic approach implemented most frequently by occupational therapists. In the 1960s, occupational therapist Dr. A. Jean Ayres introduced sensory integration—rooted in neuroscience and well ahead of its time, considering our current knowledge of neurological processes. Ayres (1979) defined *sensory integration* as the "process of organizing sensory inputs so that the brain produces a useful body response and also useful perceptions, emotions, and thoughts" (p. 28). Sensory integration theory allows therapists to explain observable behaviors of people with sensory integration challenges, plan treatment and goals, and predict therapy outcomes (Reynolds et al., 2017) for the clients with whom they work.

A drilled-down definition of sensory integration is our ability to demonstrate appropriate responses to motor and behavioral stimuli (Kilroy et al., 2019). In this feedback loop, we take sensory information from the environment, process it in our brain, and then act on or respond to it. It happens 24/7, mostly without us thinking much about it—like touching a hot stove burner and quickly removing our hand to avoid being burned. This important feedback loop is relatively seamless when our sensory systems are in sync. We are regulated. As we shared before, for most of us, our sensory systems are well integrated.

However, that is not the case for some children and adults. Because their sensory systems do not work in sync, they either crave or avoid sensory stimuli to help them get through their days. It is like an almost-empty cup for someone who craves sensory input and cannot get enough of it or an overflowing cup for someone who cannot tolerate much input. *It is truly overwhelming to be out of sync.*

Sensory processing disorder, which used to be referred to as sensory integrative disorder, occurs when the nervous system is unable to effectively take in, process, and respond to internal and environmental stimuli. Ayres (1979) referred to sensory processing disorder as a "neurological traffic jam" that stops certain parts of

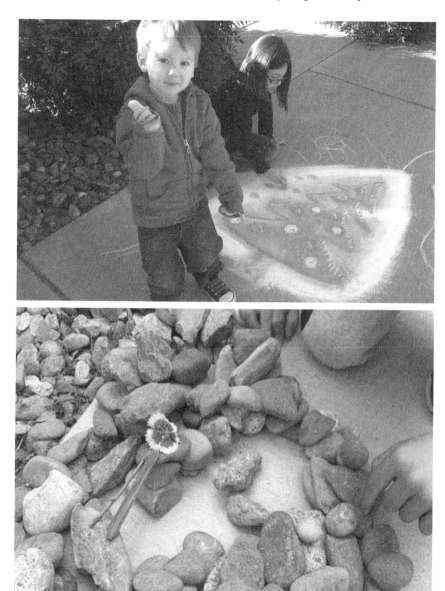

FIGURE 5.6 Creative play outdoors can take on different forms. Credit- author and Katherine Lewis.

the brain from properly taking in the information it needs to process and respond to a sensory stimulus. These challenges lead to atypical perceptions of sensation, affecting participation in daily life—like needing to wear socks inside out to avoid the sensation of the seams rubbing against your toes.

There is also a connection between sensory integration and learning. Learning depends on the brain's ability to receive and process sensory input from the environment and then plan and organize behavioral responses to that input (Bundy et al., 2002, p. 5). In the hot burner example, we need to learn quickly not to repeat the same mistake and touch a hot burner again. A key facet of sensory integration theory is that the brain has the *plasticity* to change based on experiences, good and bad, and this change influences function and behavior (Lane et al., 2019). In other words, play spaces, particularly inclusive[+] ones, must be designed to provide a wide range of sensory experiences to help children integrate their sensory systems.

At its most extreme, children with sensory processing disorder may avoid or seek out specific activities or demonstrate anxiety, distress, and anger. Some examples of sensory issues include (South Shore Therapies, n.d.):

- Hypersensitivity: avoiding certain food textures, sounds, smells, movement, and touch
- Hyposensitivity: an intense desire to take in excessive sensory experience, such as swinging, crashing, and spinning
- Notably high or low activity levels: the person cannot move enough or is reluctant to move at all
- Clumsiness or coordination issues: falling and balance issues
- Learning: difficulties fastening clothes or using pencils and scissors
- Organizational issues: difficulties staying on task or dealing with failure and increased frustration
- Poor sense of self: the person may appear lazy, unmotivated, and uninterested in engaging in challenging tasks

Sensory Integration Terminology

In this section, we provide common terminology associated with sensory integration you might come across in your work or study and want to know more about and consider when designing inclusive outdoor sensory play and learning spaces.

Sensory Processing

Sensory processing is the interaction between a person's neurological functioning and environment (Dean et al., 2018). Imagine that the weather is hot, and a water feature is within arm's reach—splashing in the water to cool off is an example of sensory processing.

Sensory Modulation

Sensory modulation is the regulatory part of sensory processing. Filtering sensory input is hard for someone with sensory modulation challenges. If they are overly sensitive to sensory input, they might live in a state of heightened emotional re-activity and apprehension toward incoming sensory stimuli, fearing it may harm them (Champagne et al., 2010). There is a strong relationship between poor sensory modulation and mental health issues. Refusing to climb the ladder to a play structure for fear of falling is an example of a sensory modulation challenge.

Sensory Defensiveness

An "over-orientation [heightened reaction] to sensory input," sensory defensiveness results from deficiencies in the modulation mechanisms of the central nervous system (Stagnitti et al., 2002, p. 178). A defensive response would be refusing sandbox play because the sand feels so rough against your skin that it is painful.

Self-regulation

Self-regulation refers to maintaining and controlling one's behaviors and emotions. An integrated sensory system contributes to self-regulation. If a tag at the back of your shirt is scratchy, you will most likely attempt to wiggle your neck and shoulders to release the sensation and move on with your day. Or you may cut off the tag or ask someone to do it for you and be done with it. However, an example of a lack of self-regulation is if the tag is bothering you so much that you cry, scream, or similarly react—and cannot articulate that the tag is causing tremendous anxiety and discomfort. Controlling your behavior and emotions is nearly impossible when the tag is completely bothersome. It may take an observant caregiver, teacher, or therapist to realize that the *tag* caused the outburst. Happily, many clothing manufacturers now print their labels directly onto most shirts, so there is no need for tags. (This is a good example of environmental sustainability—using fewer materials to convey the same amount of information.)

Sensory Registration

Sensory registration is noticing or registering sensory stimuli. Someone with sensory-registration issues may not spot things that others typically notice; they may not register the sound of honking Canada geese or, paying no attention, they might touch a hot slide.

Sensory Discrimination

Sensory discrimination entails taking in information from the environment to gain perceptual awareness (Ayres, 1972). Examples affect being aware of where the body is in space and planning movement patterns, such as navigating uneven terrain on a wooded path while staying upright on the trail or avoiding bramble and sharp overhanging branches without much effort.

What It Looks Like

Children with sensory processing and integration challenges often experience extreme difficulties participating in typical childhood activities, such as making and playing with friends, schoolwork, sports, and family interactions (Bodison & Parham, 2018; Reynolds et al., 2017). One key feature of children with sensory processing and integration challenges is their difficulty taking in accurate cues from their body when engaged in an activity (Reynolds et al., 2017). They might be unable to sit in a chair or swing without falling off, or they might not discriminate the just-right grip pressure to use when holding a paper or hard plastic cup (both examples of proprioception issues). Low muscle tone and limited core strength are also characteristics associated with sensory processing and integration. These can limit children's abilities to engage in play and self-care activities effectively (Reynolds et al., 2017). Beyond the poor body cues, low muscle tone, and decreased core strength, many children with sensory challenges cannot count on previous experiences to help them in their current situation; they fall off the chair or swing and inadvertently crush the paper cup time after time.

A Glimpse into Sensory Integration Therapy

As mentioned, occupational therapists (historically and currently) are the primary facilitators of sensory-integration-focused therapy. Increasingly, evidence is showing that the therapy is effective. On the surface, the therapy may look like unstructured gross-motor free play with scooters, swings, trampolines, ball pits, climbing, zip lines, and other fun apparatuses (to name just a few pieces of equipment used in sensory integration therapy). However, that is far from the case. Engaging with these types of motor elements in a clinical way that is grounded in evidence is the essence of the therapy. Sensory integration therapy provides children with opportunities to receive necessary and controlled sensory input that enables them to regulate their responses to sensory input and feel more secure in their interactions with their environment (Kilroy et al., 2019). Ayres believed that improved sensory integration would occur for the child receiving sensory-integration-focused therapy because participation in increasingly complex activities that are meaningful to them would lead to enhanced learning and behavior (Bundy et al., 2002).

If free play on its own improved sensory integration, there would be no need for therapy. Children with sensory processing issues would solve their own problems. Here is how the sensory integration therapy process unfolds: After establishing the baseline level of the child's skills, challenges, and functioning through extensive standardized testing and clinical observation, the occupational therapist develops an individualized treatment plan. Families may be involved with the treatment through home programs (often involving outdoor activities) to carry over the work done at the clinic. These programs are often referred to as sensory diets or sensory lifestyles. Sensory integration treatment is individualized to the child's needs but grounded in play at a level that is not too difficult for the child. The level ensures the child will not fail, nor is it so easy that the child will become bored and lack the motivation to participate or try their best. This trifecta—(1) an individualized play-based treatment (2) at a just-right level of challenge (3) that keeps the child interested—leads to adaptive responses (maintaining or improving task performance) because of changes in brain structure (Lane et al., 2019). The result of sensory integration therapy is understood to be the brain's capacity to change in response to environmental experiences (Reynolds et al., 2010).

Therapy sessions most often take place inside therapy clinics. They are set up to provide the child with structure and freedom, encouraging "constructive exploration" (South Shore Therapies, n.d.). Through this careful balance of structure and freedom, the child's neural organization and sense of self develops. As the child progresses through increasingly complex activities—at their own pace—the therapist withdraws some structure and encourages the child to take control of the session and, in time, to take command of their life.

A Sensory Way to Improve Outdoor Play Space Quality and Diversity

For the sake of the sensory systems, planning and design matter! Sensory overload can lead to or increase stress and anxiety, regardless of whether someone has sensory processing challenges (Martin et al., 2019). Sensory under- or overload affects the ways we interact with our social and natural or built environments. Providing the just-right balance—reducing or increasing sensory input from the environment—can support participation in daily activities. Too much or too little input may result in a child (or adult) being unable to do what they want or need to do—play, learn, work, or take care of themselves (Reynolds et al., 2017). A well-designed outdoor play environment that balances sensory elements, providing alerting and calming experiences, enables children to seek them out, better process sensory input, and, in turn, self-regulate. You may recall that self-regulation is being able to control emotions and behaviors, a skill necessary to play, learn, and perform daily self-care tasks like dressing, bathing, grooming, eating, and later, work and engage in leisure activities. Self-regulation is important—and an integrated sensory system positively contributes to regulation (see Figure 5.7).

Integrating sensory features into outdoor play spaces supports inclusivity. For example, colorful, textured play panels expand exploratory play opportunities. They provide abundant sensory and learning experiences, such as counting and identifying colors while exploring the panels by touch and sight. Designing and installing these same panels—but of varying sizes, shapes, and colors and at different heights—even more robustly supports inclusive[+] play at all levels while affording flexibility in accessing the feature, such as by hand, arm, head, trunk, leg, or foot. The learning experience that has always been a part of play, whether or not obvious, can now be expanded to include categorizing by size and shape

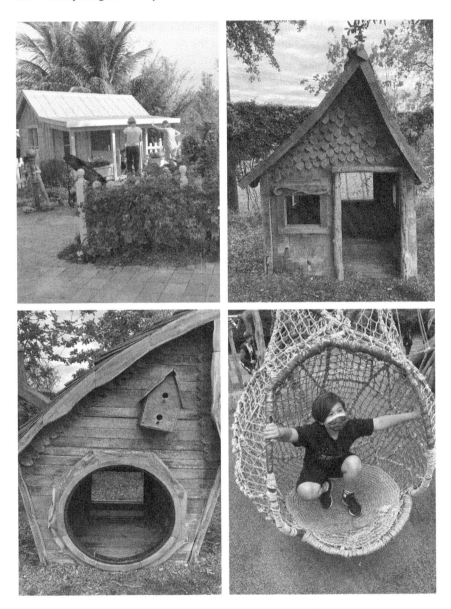

FIGURE 5.7 Cozy spaces for refuge and self-regulation. Credit- author.

while touching and looking at the panels. Outdoor chimes that are equally usable from seated or standing positions and activated by mallets or hands benefit all children at play. They can touch, hear, move, and look. Motion-detection devices require little physical effort to trigger features like sound or light elements that activate when children walk or roll by them. Color changes in the play equipment or pathways provide perceptible visual information for elevation changes, assist with navigation, and delineate pathways and play areas. These may help children who prefer solitary play or benefit from quieter play.

Designing inclusive[+] outdoor play spaces with a sensory focus, in collaboration with occupational therapists, can lead to more spontaneous play. When done well, these spaces can become outdoor therapy clinics where occupational, physical, speech and language, and recreational therapists take their clients outside for therapy. When you think about it, isn't it better to have therapy "in the real world" and practice real-life skills where they naturally occur than in a clinic? Let's keep talking about this idea.

Collaborative Design

We hope that, by now, you see the value of an interdisciplinary process combining landscape architecture with occupational therapy in creating the most-balanced sensory designs. This is a dream approach. It blends a deep understanding of the sensory systems, their impact on daily function, and environmental modification to improve participation from team occupational therapy with a deep understanding of landforms, preservation, sustainability, and design from the landscape architecture team.

The designer's role as part of such an interdisciplinary team is critical in transforming therapeutic strategies that occupational therapists recommend into designed elements. The outcome could be a well-designed inclusive outdoor play space or, perhaps, an actual outdoor clinic to treat children with sensory integration and processing issues. Just think of the possibilities! Collaboratively, this design approach ensures inclusion in each project of alerting sensory spaces for children who crave sensory stimuli and calming sensory spaces for children who need to retreat and rewind. All children and their families can then best nurture all eight sensory systems. This approach is important in outdoor play environments but applies to *any* designed space. It may improve children's self-regulation and behavior when adapted to support participation with carefully selected alerting and calming activities (Reynolds et al., 2017). This approach is the key to sensory integration and, more holistically, to inclusive[+] outdoor play.

Final Thoughts

We return to where we started. This chapter is not intended to be a comprehensive review of sensory integration or provide the information necessary for a designer working alone to create safe, effective, sensory-focused inclusive[+] outdoor play spaces. Unintentional errors in sensory design that lead to over- or underregistration can exacerbate existing sensory issues, something nobody wants to happen. Instead, the information in this chapter provides foundational information about sensation and sensory integration to engage with occupational therapists and design together the most effective, engaging, and sought-after outdoor play spaces that nourish and enrich children's sensory systems and enable them to do what is most important—have fun and be their happiest selves.

BOX 5.1 CASE STUDY: ELS FOR AUTISM SENSORY ARTS GARDEN (FIGURES 5.8–5.10)

Project Information:

Name
Els for Autism Sensory Arts Garden

Designer
Dirtworks Landscape Architecture, PC

Location
Jupiter, FL

Size
1,207 m² or 0.3 acre

Year Built
2017 completed

Age Group
3–21 years

Description:

The Sensory Arts Garden at the Els Center of Excellence was designed for individuals with autism and the caregivers, educators, and therapists who support them. It is located on the 26-acre campus of the Els Center of Excellence in Palm Beach County, Florida. The goal of the project was to create an inclusive, sensory-rich therapeutic environment with places of refuge that support individuals with autism and enhance their capacity to work, play, socialize, and learn. The garden offers users choices in how it can be experienced. It contains active spaces for gardening, a group-activity area, two learning spaces, places to seek quiet and self-regulate, two small water features and a large water wall to interact with, musical instruments, and graded "places away," which are nook-like areas that provide opportunities for different levels of socialization and sensory enrichment. This small refuge balances alerting and calming sensory experiences to allay anxiety and enrich the senses through its high level of consistency and repetition.

Websites:

- https://www.elsforautism.org/the-els-center-of-excellence/sensory-arts-garden/
- https://dirtworks.us/portfolio/sensory-arts-garden-els-center-excellence/

Traditional Inclusive Features	Inclusive⁺ Features
• Accessible path of travel • Strong, durable materials for planters, seating, tables, entry structures, swings	• Smooth, consistent tinted concrete paving surfaces reduce glare and add a level of predictability to the garden • Curved paths and designed elements eliminate awkward corners and address potential collisions and adverse reactions

(Continued)

- Varied-height planters for seated and standing access
- Wheelchair access seating at activity tables
- Natural shade options
- 100% at-grade; no slopes
- Clear site lines throughout the garden
- Varied seating options

- Considerations for routine, consistent patterns, sightlines, and wayfinding allow continued discovery, autonomy, and flexible use
- Highly comprehensible: easy transitions and clear circulation patterns and destinations
- Transitional spaces to welcome individuals into the garden offer a place to pause before entering and take in unobstructed views of the entire garden
- "Sensory rooms," centrally aligned within the garden feature, are easily accessed custom planters filled with engaging, safe, sensory appropriate plants
- Planting strategy was deliberately shaped through a melding of health-promoting design principles and considerations for the unique needs of individuals with autism
- A series of reduced and integrated sensory spaces, or "places away," along the garden perimeter provide calming counterpoints for those who may experience hypersensitivity or wish to seek a moment of respite and refuge
- Planting palettes within "places away" are purposely muted to enhance feelings of serenity and tranquility
- Pebble paving, individually selected to conform to the curvature of small feet, enhances balance, tactile engagement, and gross-motor skills
- Varied seating types, social and solitary: structured, trunk-supporting, straight-backed benches with armrests provide comfort in key areas
- Pebble seats in different shapes and contours offer a playful alternative and varying levels of proprioceptive and vestibular experiences
- Small, movable musical elements activate the various rooms with sound

Remarks:

In establishing a vibrant outdoor living classroom, an enriching therapeutic environment, and an inclusive welcoming space for all, the Sensory Arts Garden

(Continued)

advances the Els Center of Excellence's position as a leader in the field. It broadens their influence within the autism community and promotes the value, acceptance, and inclusion of individuals with autism. The inclusive+ garden extends invitations for children and young adults to feel whole and safe on their own terms—to be part of something bigger than themselves without feeling overwhelmed. Since opening in 2017, individuals with autism have found reprieve in the garden's "places away" and enrichment by exploring the plants in the sensory rooms. Students identify favorite spots within the garden and return to engage with these spaces daily, exploring their subtle changes and new growth. The garden has become an established space for outdoor instruction, providing opportunities to connect with students who may be challenging to reach. Music and yoga classes and reading groups all benefit from this sensory-rich living classroom that welcomes all, regardless of age, ability, background, or preference. Within a lush and safe setting, the garden provides opportunities and choices for each visitor to engage with nature on their own terms, in their own way, and at their own pace.

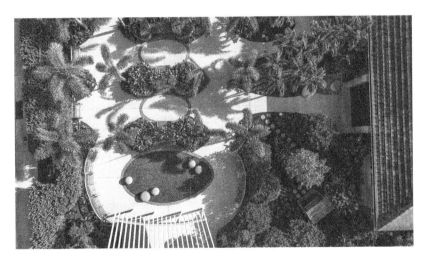

FIGURE 5.8   Bird's eye view. Credit- Robin Hill.

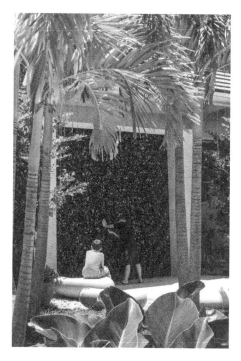

FIGURE 5.9 The wall of water is an engaging multisensory experience. Credit- Mark Tepper.

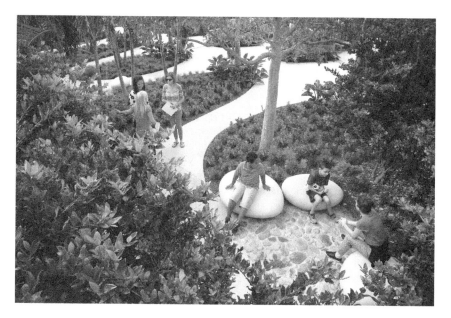

FIGURE 5.10 Places away in the garden provide opportunities to self-regulate and make choices. Credit- Robin Hill.

References

Ayres, A. J. (1972). Treatment of sensory integrative dysfunction. *Australian Journal of Occupational Therapy, 19*(2), 88. https://doi.org/10.1111/j.1440-1630.1972.tb00547.x

Ayres, A. J. (1979). *Sensory integration and the child.* Western Psychological Services.

Bennie, M. (2016, March 7). *What is interoception and how does it impact those with autism?* Autism Awareness Centre. https://autismawarenesscentre.com/what-is-interoception-and-how-does-it-impact-autism/

Ben-Sasson, A., Carter, A. S., & Briggs-Gowan, M. J. (2009). Sensory over-responsivity in elementary school: Prevalence and social–emotional correlates. *Journal of Abnormal Child Psychology, 37*, 705–716. https://doi.org/10.1007/s10802-008-9295-8

Bodison, S. C., & Parham, L. D. (2018). Specific sensory techniques and sensory environmental modifications for children and youth with sensory integration difficulties: A systematic review. *American Journal of Occupational Therapy, 72*(1), 7201190040p1–7201190040p11. https://doi.org/10.5014/ajot.2018.029413

Bundy, A. C., Lane, S. J., & Murray, E. A. (2002). *Sensory integration: Theory and practice.* F.A. Davis.

Bushdid, C., Magnasco, M. O., Vosshall, L. B., & Keller, A. (2014). Humans can discriminate more than 1 trillion olfactory stimuli. *Science, 343*(6177), 1370–1372. https://doi.org/10.1126/science.1249168

Champagne, T., Koomar, J., & Olson, L. (2010). Sensory processing, evaluation, and intervention in mental health. *Occupational Therapy Practice, 15*(5), CE1–CE8.

Craig, A. D. (2015). *How do you feel? An interoceptive moment with your neurobiological self.* Princeton University Press.

Curley, A. M. (2015, January 27). *Making sense of scents: Smell and the brain.* BrainFacts.org. https://www.brainfacts.org/thinking-sensing-and-behaving/smell/2015/making-sense-of-scents-smell-and-the-brain

Dean, E. E., Little, L., Tomchek, S., & Dunn, W. (2018). Sensory processing in the general population: Adaptability, resiliency, and challenging behavior. *American Journal of Occupational Therapy, 72*(1), 7201195060p1–7201195060p8. https://doi.org/10.5014/ajot.2018.019919

Khalsa, S. S., & Lapidus, R. C. (2016). Can interoception improve the pragmatic search for biomarkers in psychiatry? *Frontiers in Psychiatry, 7*, Article 121. https://doi.org/10.3389/fpsyt.2016.00121

Kilroy, E., Aziz-Zadeh, L., & Cermak, S. (2019). Ayres theories of autism and sensory integration revisited: What contemporary neuroscience has to say. *Brain Sciences, 9*(3), Article 68. https://doi.org/10.3390/brainsci9030068

Lane, S. J., Mailloux, Z., Schoen, S., Bundy, A., May-Benson, T. A., Parham, L. D., Smith Roley, S., & Schaaf, R. C. (2019). Neural foundations of Ayres Sensory Integration®. *Brain Sciences, 9*(7), Article 153. https://doi.org/10.3390/brainsci9070153

Lobe. (n.d.). *How does the auditory system work?* [Online blog post]. Lobe. https://www.lobe.ca/en/blog/protect-my-hearing/Auditory-system-works

Martin, N., Milton, D. E. M., Krupa, J., Brett, S., Bulman, K., Callow, D., Copeland, F., Cunningham, L., Ellis, W., Harvey, T., Moranska, M., Roach, R., & Wilmot, S. (2019). The sensory school: Working with teachers, parents and pupils to create good sensory conditions. *Advances in Autism, 5*(2), 131–140. https://doi.org/10.1108/AIA-09-2018-0034

Merriam-Webster. (n.d.). *Merriam-Webster.com dictionary.* http://www.merriam-webster.com/dictionary/sensation

National Eye Institute. (2022, June 10). *Refractive errors.* https://www.nei.nih.gov/learn-about-eye-health/eye-conditions-and-diseases/refractive-errors#:~:text=Did%20you%20know%3F,that%20can%20cause%20blurry%20vision

Pfeiffer, B., May-Benson, T. A., & Bodison, S. C. (2018). State of the science of sensory integration research with children and youth. *American Journal of Occupational Therapy, 72*, 7201170010p1–7201170010p4. https://doi.org/10.5014/ajot.2018.721003

Price, C. J., & Hooven, C. (2018). Interoceptive awareness skills for emotion regulation: Theory and approach of mindful awareness in body-oriented therapy (MABT). *Frontiers in Psychology, 9*, 798. https://doi.org/10.3389/fpsyg.2018.00798

Price, C. J., & Remington, L. A. (2012). *Clinical anatomy and physiology of the visual system* (3rd ed.). Butterworth Heinemann.

Raising an Extraordinary Person. (n.d.). *The tactile system.* https://hes-extraordinary.com/the-tactile-system

Reynolds, S., Glennon, T. J., Ausderau, K., Bendixen, R. M., Kuhaneck, H. M., Pfeiffer, B., Watling, R., Wilkinson, K., & Bodison, S. C. (2017). Using a multifaceted approach to working with children who have differences in sensory processing and integration. *American Journal of Occupational Therapy, 71*, 7102360010p1–710236001p10. https://doi.org/10.5014/ajot.2017.019281

Reynolds, S., Lane, S. J., & Richards, L. (2010). Using animal models of enriched environments to inform research on sensory integration intervention for the rehabilitation of neurodevelopmental disorders. *Journal of Neurodevelopmental Disorders, 2*, 120–132. https://doi.org/10.1007/s11689-010-9053-4

Sincero, S. M. (2013, March 18). *The visual system.* Explorable. https://explorable.com/visual-system-en

South Shore Therapies. (n.d.). *Sensory integration therapy.* https://southshoretherapies.com/services/sensory-integration

SPD Australia. (n.d.a.). *The olfactory system.* https://spdaustralia.com.au/the-olfactory-system/

SPD Australia. (n.d.b.). *The prorioceptive system.* https://spdaustralia.com.au/the-proprioceptive-system/

Stagnitti, K., Raison, P., & Ryan, P. (2002). Sensory defensiveness syndrome: A paediatric perspective and case study. *Australian Journal of Occupational Therapy, 46*, 175–187. https://doi.org/10.1046/j.1440-1630.1999.00197.x

Star Institute. (n.d.). *Your 8 senses.* https://www.spdstar.org/basic/your-8-senses#f5.

6

INCLUSIVE DESIGN

Introduction

Play is a social process, and opportunities included in play should be available to every child. Not only should it be *available*, according to Article 31 of the UN Convention on the Rights of the Child, "*Every* [emphasis added] child has the right to . . . engage in play and recreational activities" (UNICEF, 2012). All too often, though, planning efforts relate mainly to mobility impairments. These efforts overshadow the need for a more comprehensive approach focused on understanding children with other types of visible and invisible disabilities and identifying developmentally appropriate risk levels in play for these children.

Globally, UNICEF (2021) estimated that nearly 240 million children are identified as having disabilities. Their report also found that in measures of well-being, children with disabilities are more disadvantaged and marginalized than their peers without disabilities. In the United States, the percentage of children identified with all types of disabilities rose from 3.9% to 4.3% between 2008 and 2019 (U.S. Census Bureau, 2021). Although cognitive disabilities are most common among children 5 years or older, other disabilities for that age group include motor and physical sensory, social-emotional disabilities, and chronic conditions like cancer, diabetes, and obesity (Christensen & Jeon, 2006). This information is important because it demonstrates the increased identification of children with various types of disabilities, all of whom have the need and right to play and engage in recreation in ways that are meaningful for them.

Disability in the context of play is often mistakenly understood as a child's inability to experience the play environment because of limitations from their impairment. Defining disability in this way—putting the onus on the child's condition—usually results in attempts to fix the child's impairment rather than the play

DOI: 10.4324/9781003193890-6

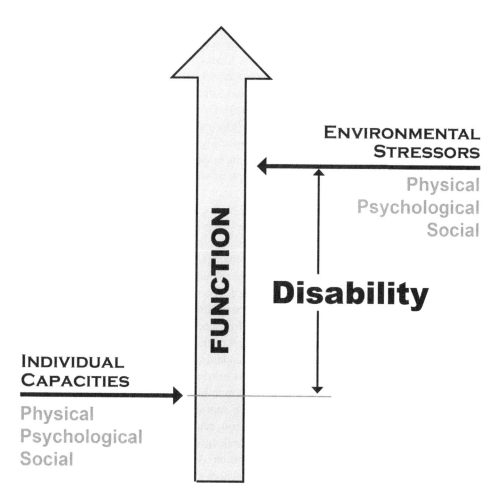

FIGURE 6.1 Personal and environmental factors that influence function. Credit- Adapted
from: Aslaksen et al. (1997).

environment. In reality, the environments we occupy and engage with can and do limit children from participating in play (Brown et al., 2021). This inequity represents both environmental and occupational injustices, the negative effects of which cannot be underestimated (see Figure 6.1).

This paradigm to fix the disability rather than the environment results in a lack of societal understanding of the need for facilities and outdoor environments that are truly accessible. These environments should meet the needs of people across a wide range of disabilities, whether visible (e.g., cerebral palsy or limb loss) or not (e.g., learning disability, asthma, or mental illness; Prellwitz & Skär, 2007). It is often the invisible disabilities that design overlooks (Brown et al., 2021). In fact, 14 million people in the United Kingdom have disabilities, but 70% of those disabilities are invisible (Kelly & Mutebi, 2023). Of the 42 million Americans with disabilities, 96% have invisible disabilities (Morgan, 2020)—meaning that designing only or primarily for individuals with mobility issues does not effectively address the issue of what fully accessible or inclusive[+] play space design is. In this chapter, we introduce the origin and concepts of what we consider inclusive[+] play space design to be.

We estimate that hundreds of inclusive play spaces are under construction or have been built throughout the world, and happily, many children enjoy them. However, somewhere during the design process, the core intentions and purposes for creating spaces where *all* children and their families could play often get lost in the details of laws and regulations. These include the ADA (1990) regulations, ASTM safety standards, "Canadian Standards Association Standard for Children's Playspaces and Equipment, and Australian Standards, AS 4685, Playground Equipment and Surfacing, and AS 1428, Design for Access and Mobility" (Brown et al., 2021, p. 3). Equipment selections and budget restrictions also must be considered.

However, although these regulations, standards, and the like are extremely important, they are only part of the picture. As previously mentioned, the disproportionate focus on the needs of children with mobility challenges far too frequently overshadows the need for a comprehensive approach that truly represents inclusive[+] design for social and emotional inclusion, neurodiversity, sensory regulation, graduating levels of physical and mental challenges, cognitive simplicity, and ample opportunities for discovery and exploration. As Christensen and Jeon (2006) suggested, comprehensive inclusive[+] play spaces are most effective when created with an activity-based approach founded on evidence-based design. Let's explore the possibilities.

Refocusing Design

The wonderful web of play involves more than a child and their interaction and engagement with the environment. Directly or indirectly, caregivers, families, siblings, grandparents, and peers also influence play. Accordingly, design must reflect an even broader conceptualization of what inclusive[+] play spaces incorporate. A recent focus on evidence-based design has led to a deeper understanding of what the term *inclusive* means. We think of it as the integration between childhood development and play-related research findings, particularly findings focused on children with disabilities.

The outcome of these findings generates outdoor recreational and play spaces that transcend the traditional and introduce a new form of play. Research continues across the world for a better understanding of social behaviors and how children interact with outdoor environments and those around them (Hazlehurst et al., 2022; Johnstone et al., 2022). The principles of inclusive[+] play space design described in this chapter are based on academic research and observations of research put into practice.

When planning or designing play spaces, keep in mind that a comprehensive, interdisciplinary team approach based on evidence-based knowledge of the needs of children with and without disabilities is required. This knowledge includes understanding that risk tolerance for differing ability levels can improve the success of the play spaces and lead to well-used outdoor environments that children of *all* abilities will enjoy. Again, we highlight the need for inclusive[+] play spaces for the health and well-being of all children and their caregivers.

Inclusive[+] Design

We chose to display the evolution of inclusive design with a "+" symbol after the term to highlight that what we are presenting does not stop at the traditional use of the word *inclusive*. Instead, the term is expanded to incorporate recent evidence-based research that includes a greater understanding of how environmental and sensory experiences, as well as stress and trauma, affect overall childhood development.

Written by occupational therapist and neuroscientist Dr. A. Jean Ayres, *Sensory Integration and the Child* was a landmark publication for pediatric health care providers, educators, and caregivers. Ayres developed sensory integration theory in the 1950s. With the publication of her book two decades later, in 1979, she provided long-sought answers and an explanation to frustrated caregivers who could not understand their children's behaviors or how it seemed to negatively affect their overall development and capacity to learn. The sensory integration framework became a beacon for therapists (particularly occupational therapists), educators, and even physicians to use in developing intervention plans that help these children better function and participate in daily life. Although designers are not trained to facilitate sensory integration therapies, a basic understanding of the theory is critically important for decision-making when designing inclusive[+] outdoor play spaces. (Please refer to Chapter 5, "Sensory Integration: Why It Matters," for more detailed information about sensory integration.)

Experiencing enduring childhood stress and trauma is understood to negatively affect all aspects of childhood development (Smith & Pollak, 2020). Play is a normative part of childhood (Stenman et al., 2019); as such, it can help reduce the impact of stress and trauma. Because access to nature is associated with reduced stress and improved mental health (Mygind et al., 2019), play that is grounded in nature can help children self-regulate their emotions and experience internal balance (LaPiere & Dion, 2022). There is increasing interest in trauma-responsive design. Working alongside trained allied and mental health professionals, landscape designers can play a vital role in creating inclusive[+] outdoor play spaces that meet a wide range of children's needs but mostly for children with a history of stress and trauma.

Introducing Inclusive[+] Play Space Design

Recall that the evolution of play underwent a slow trajectory over the recent decades. An increased understanding of childhood development, mental and physical health, and disabilities propelled this evolution forward. Design is continually improving, in part because of a greater understanding of the importance of play and the need to support play opportunities for children with visible and invisible health conditions in outdoor environments. This understanding provides vital insight into how creating recreational spaces for children and families can become progressively better and more inclusive. A readily available diversity of choice and activity approach encourages many positive outcomes, including developmentally appropriate independent play away from caregivers. This is a significant and sought-after outcome of inclusive[+] play space design.

The only way many children with disabilities might play and interact with peers is with help from caregivers. Needing help from an adult caregiver to play with peers can be embarrassing or just, unfortunately, what is necessary to engage in play. Hands-on assistance with play limits the children's chances to explore risk, make their own choices, and experience heightened self-esteem and confidence (Goodley & Runswick-Cole, 2010; Graham et al., 2015; Mather, 1981; Van Melik & Althuizen, 2022) (see Figure 6.2).

The timeline shown in Figure 6.3 provides a brief snapshot of some major historic legislative actions, research, and publications that led to the current play space design trends. This timeline is not intended to be a comprehensive study of the history of inclusive[+] play space design but rather a summary of critical milestones that shaped our current approach.

The Roots of Inclusive[+] Play Space Design

Inclusive[+] play originates from a design trend that emerged in the late 1990s and early 2000s termed *accessible play*. The concept of accessible play was a direct result of the passage of the ADA (1990). Significant attention was brought to the fact that ADA codes established by the Federal government in no way addressed children's play spaces. The "accessible play movement" began as a result of this omission. An early nonprofit social enterprise called Boundless Play paved the way for the movement; by 2009, this organization had helped build 190 accessible play

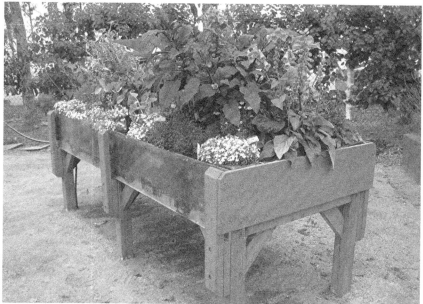

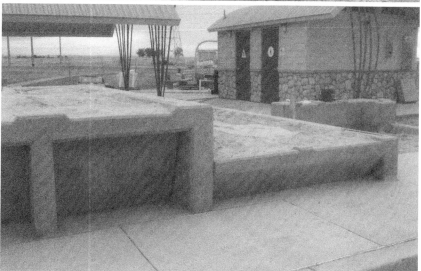

FIGURE 6.2 Inclusive options for children to independently garden and play with sand. Credit- author.

spaces (Right to Play, 2022). The focus of the Boundless Play movement was to make play spaces more accessible for children with physical and mobility impairments by bringing in more ramp structures and opportunities to reach higher places in a play space. No other disabilities were considered with such a comprehensive

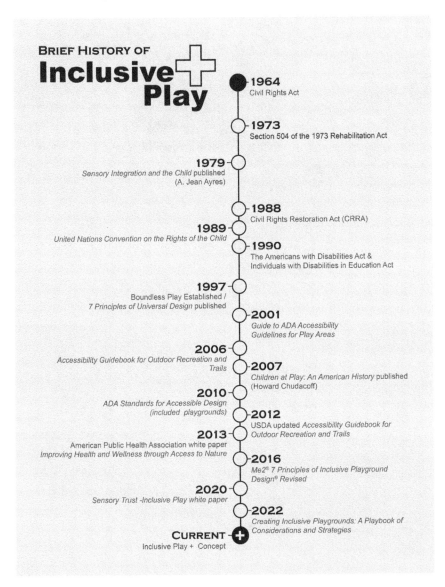

FIGURE 6.3 A timeline of inclusive⁺ play space design. Credit- author.

emphasis. Another trend soon followed: The "all-abilities play movement" attempted to improve on the accessible play concept by recognizing disabilities, such as blindness and low vision, auditory, and cognitive disabilities, and introducing a wider range of play elements.

As described in this chapter, inclusive⁺ play space design grew out of the all-abilities play movement. Designers and advocates recognized the limitations of disability-related building codes and regulations and sought ways to advocate for and address myriad other overlooked disabilities. Beyond designing for mobility, visual, auditory, and cognitive disabilities, inclusive⁺ play space design looks to meet the needs of a broader spectrum of challenges. This spectrum includes "invisible" disabilities, such as sensory processing disorders and social-emotional, developmental, and chronic health conditions (Owen et al., 2017; Patrick & Hollenbeck, 2021; Radzi et al., 2020).

Even though the design and play community uses the terms *accessible play* and *all-abilities play* interchangeably to encompass inclusion, a truly inclusive⁺ play space recognizes that disability can be visible or invisible. It also acknowledges age-related disabilities by designing and programming for all who may use and support children in play spaces (e.g., caregivers, grandparents, and siblings). Table 6.1 provides a quick guide to the conceptual differences between modern inclusive⁺ play space design and traditional accessibility.

TABLE 6.1 A Comparison of Inclusive⁺ and Accessible Play

Modern inclusive⁺ play	Traditional accessibility
Encourages social participation in play	Establishes minimum and maximum slopes and grades
Engages families in social interaction	Establishes head clearances
Provides cognitively clear, solid, and manageable surfaces	Establishes all weather surfaces (loose or unitary)
Allows for risk-taking	Establishes knee and arm clearances
Enables *all* children, families, and friends to play together at *all* elevations	Establishes a minimum number of areas/activities accessible at ground level
Provides high-quality, well-designed play environments for *all*	Ensures those with disabilities have the same right to participate
Encourages extra-wide travel paths and aisles	Establishes minimum widths of travel paths and aisles
Eliminates barriers and discourages stigmas	Highlights differences in abilities
Provides for independent choice-making	Establishes an accessible path of travel
Provides as much diversity as possible in play opportunities and experiences	Establishes minimum standards to be met
Addresses justice (fixing the system, not just tools)	Addresses equality and equity issues

* *inequality (unequal access to play)*
* *equality (evenly distributed appliances and assistance for play)*
* *equity (custom appliances and features that highlight and address inequality)*
* *justice (fixing the system/environment to offer equal access to appliances and opportunities)*

The Rehabilitation Act (1973) was signed into law in 1973 and amended in 1979. The Act stated that no person could be denied the benefits or activity within a program, activity, or project funded with federal money (https://www.ecfr.gov/current/title-49/part-27). This law served as the precursor to later legislation like the ADA (1990) and the Individuals with Disabilities in Education Act (IDEA, 2004), which forever changed the way persons with disabilities would be treated.

Although slow to fruition, the ADA (1990) and IDEA (2004) were eventually signed into law. As the first laws of their kind worldwide, they established minimum requirements for the built environment and prohibited discrimination based on disability—regardless of the origin of the funding source, municipality, or organization. This legislation included recreational areas but did not include play spaces specifically. In 2001, the *Guide to ADA Accessibility Guidelines for Play Areas* was published to fill voids in the 1990 legislation (Architectural and Transportation Barriers Compliance Board, 2000). This guide addressed many challenges families faced in play spaces, such as elevated play elements, ground-level elements, types of play equipment, age separation, accessible routes, and more.

The guidelines were updated in 2006 but—being just *guidelines*—were not enforceable until a much overdue revision to the 1990 ADA legislation was published in 2010. The *ADA Standards for Accessible Design* incorporated standards such as the required number of elevated and ground-level accessible play features, the width of access walks, transition heights, and many other play and outdoor amenities (U.S. Department of Justice, 2010). Shortly thereafter, the U.S. Department of Agriculture (2012) published an updated version of the *Accessibility Guidebook for Outdoor Recreation and Trails*. The guidebook now provides enforceable accessibility policies for national forests but serves only as guidelines for integrating accessible features, trails, and outdoor recreation areas elsewhere.

Universal and Inclusive[+] Design

Terms such as *design for all*, *barrier-free design*, *human-centered design*, *universal design*, and *inclusive design* are often used interchangeably. Regardless of the term, the intent of these concepts is "increasing the accessibility of the interactive system for the widest possible range of use" (Persson et al., 2015, p. 504). Here we focus on two design concepts—universal and inclusive[+] design—often used to describe specialized outdoor play space design. Universal and inclusive[+] design start with accessible design but call for designers' more creative and imaginative engagement in designing places, products, and technologies that will work seamlessly for the widest possible group of potential users (Institute for Human Centered Design, n.d.)—which, in this case, are children and their caregivers.

Universal Design

Universal design was developed by the late architect Ron Mace and his colleagues at North Carolina State University in 1997. Its roots emanated from the barrier-free and accessible-design approaches (Persson et al., 2015). *Universal design* is the "design of products and environments to be usable by all people, to the greatest extent possible, without the need for adaptation or specialized design" (NC State University Center for Universal Design, 1997, para. 4). Going beyond what is required by the standards set forth in the ADA (1990), universal design contains seven principles:

- Equitable use
- Flexibility in use
- Simple and intuitive use
- Perceptible information
- Tolerance for error
- Low physical effort
- Size and space for approach and use

Together, the seven principles are intended to guide the design of products, services, and environments that improve the quality of life for everyone (Table 6.2). Several research studies have focused on the positive effects of universally designed play spaces on children's physical and social-emotional health and development (Lynch et al., 2020; Moore et al., 2022; Stanton-Chapman & Schmidt, 2017).

Inclusive Design

In the United Kingdom, *inclusive design* has been the preferred term for design for all since the 1990s. As defined by the Commission for Architecture and the Built Environment (2006), "Inclusive design is about making places everyone can use. . . . It aims to remove the barriers that create undue effort and separation. It enables everyone to participate equally, confidently and independently in everyday activities" (p. 3). Products or environments are designed to place users at the heart of the design process. They acknowledge diversity and difference, offer choices to better accommodate all users, provide flexibility in how the product or environment is used, and lead to design outcomes that are convenient and enjoyable for everyone (pp. 8–15). When these principles are followed, they can lead to designs that are inclusive, responsive, convenient, accommodating, welcoming, and realistic (p. 19) (see Table 6.2).

Inclusive[+] Design

Inclusive[+] design builds upon the wisdom of universal and inclusive design and pushes its limits in the best possible ways. Beyond designing for mobility, visual, auditory, and cognitive disabilities, inclusive[+] play space design looks to meet the needs of a broader spectrum of diversity, which extends far beyond disability. To fully embrace and welcome an authentic sense of inclusion for age, cultural, gender and sexual orientation, and socioeconomics, diversity must also be considered when designing an inclusive[+] play space. As the name suggests, inclusive[+] play

TABLE 6.2 Comparing the Relationship Between Universal and Inclusive Design Principles

Universal design	Inclusive design
Equitable use. The design is useful and marketable to people with diverse abilities.	**Inclusive.** The design can be used safely, easily, and with dignity. **Welcoming.** The design presents no disabling barriers that might exclude some people.
Flexibility in use. The design accommodates a wide range of individual preferences and abilities.	**Realistic.** The design offers more than one solution to help balance everyone's needs and recognizes that one solution may not work for all. **Responsive.** The design considers what people say they need and want; it is flexible so different people can use the space in different ways.
Simple and intuitive. Use of the design is easy to understand regardless of the user's experience, knowledge, language skills, or current concentration level.	**Convenient.** Everyone can use the design without too much effort or separation.
Perceptible information. The design effectively communicates necessary information to the user, regardless of ambient conditions or user's sensory abilities.	**Accommodating.** The design accommodates all people, regardless of age, gender, mobility, ethnicity, or circumstances.
Tolerance for error. The design minimizes hazards and adverse consequences of accidental or unintended actions.	**Inclusive.** The design can be used safely, easily, and with dignity.
Low physical effort. The design can be used efficiently, comfortably, and with minimum fatigue.	**Convenient.** Everyone can use the design without too much effort or separation.
Size and space for approach and use. The design provides appropriate size and space for approach, reach, manipulation, and use, regardless of the user's body size, posture, or mobility.	**Accommodating.** The design accommodates all people, regardless of age, gender, mobility, ethnicity, or circumstances.

Source: Adapted from: Commission for Architecture and the Built Environment (2006); NC State University Center for Universal Design (1997).

spaces reflect opportunities for all children to engage in various play typologies. The space itself enables children to experience risk at their tolerance; be creative, social, and independent; and engage in multisensory experiences that best suit them. Features such as gender-neutral restrooms; listening and immersive engagement sessions with relevant key stakeholders to help understand the local culture and incorporate elements of it into the play space through art, plantings, and interactive features; installing information kiosks with multilanguage information to direct visitors to local social services; and hosting key social service events in the play space are other strategies to help achieve an inclusive⁺ play space.

Principles of Inclusive⁺ Play Space Design

As described in this chapter, many universal and inclusive design principles reflect effective designs for all types of inclusive spaces, including implementation in the physical play space environment. The following discussion expands the conversation about the physical environment and focuses on social considerations—the play typologies we explored in Chapter 3, "History and Value of Outdoor Play." When incorporated into play space design, each typology helps create diverse and inclusive play spaces and opportunities that meet a wide variety of needs for children and their families.

Independent Play

While on summer vacation in the greater Chicago area with my (Chad) family several years ago, we made a late-morning visit to a local neighborhood park. I was amazed at the lack of maintenance and the number of hazardous conditions. Metal wires showed through worn rope climbers, play-structure ramps suddenly ended where paths once were, only remnants of safety surfacing could be found on the soil surface, and many pieces of equipment were rusted with age. During this visit, I became one of the "helicopter parents" so widely criticized in society. As I recognized the dangers in the play area, an innate response emerged—prompting me to help the children navigate the environment so they could identify and avoid the hazards. Although I needed to be involved for my children's safety in this instance, I am a huge proponent of allowing their independent choices and risk (but not harm) in play spaces.

This reasoning comes from understanding that independent play is one experience in which children have chances to learn skills that will support independence, such as decision-making, confidence, self-reliance, and resilience (Murniyati & Wardhani, 2023; Sunarty & Dirawan Darma, 2015). On a macro level, play spaces designed as safe and comfortable places offer inherent opportunities to support independent thinking. Children can be given chances to learn the consequences, good and bad, of the decisions they make. Caregivers can feel comfortable letting those natural decisions and consequences occur for children of all abilities. Independent play features might include loose parts and multiple access points to a play structure (e.g., ramps, steps, climbing wall, nets).

Caregivers and safety organizations are often criticized for not giving children space to trip, fall, get hurt, and learn for themselves. What would happen if caregivers were discouraged from participating in or even prohibited from supervised play spaces, and children were left to their own devices to experience independent play? Would it be the child's fault if they played on and were hurt in an unsafe play space designed by adults? These are questions to consider, particularly as they overlay with risky play.

Physical and Risky Play

Risky play is exhilarating and thrilling (Obee et al., 2021), and risky outdoor play benefits children's healthy development (Gray, 2020). It helps them manage stress, learn to follow through with an activity, improve social interaction skills, increase creativity, learn about human fragility, understand their limitations, recognize areas for improvement, and form positive, proactive attitudes toward others and the environment (Brussoni et al., 2012; Coates & Pimlott-Wilson, 2019; Gleave, 2008; Tai, 2022). Other developmental benefits of risky play include improved motor skills and cognitive awareness of the environment (Sandseter, 2009).

Through her extensive research, Dr. Ellen Sandseter, a professor of early childhood education in Norway, identified categories of risk in which children engage. These categories include

1) Play with great heights. These types of risky play involve climbing and jumping from elevated surfaces—trees, poles, rocks, play climbers, hills or anything else, as long as the opportunity to climb or jump is there. . . 2) Play with high speed; spinning or riding bikes, scooters, etc. down steep ramps or hills. . .3) Play with harmful tools; hammers, saws, nails, sharp objects. . . 4) Play near dangerous elements; running water, tree limbs, crevasses. . . 5) Rough-and-tumble play; physical contact and. . .x 6) Play where the children can "disappear"/ get lost; places to hide.

(Sandseter, 2007, pp. 243–248)

Partly because development is uneven—for example, children's cognitive and decision-making skills are not as refined as their motor skills—it is not uncommon to see risky play unfold in unexpected ways. In scenarios where the children's motor skills exceed their thinking skills, risky play can manifest in utilizing manufactured play space equipment and natural elements in the play space in ways they were not intended to be used. These might entail jumping from high places and platforms, climbing structures or trees, and mock aggression (Sandseter, 2009). The degree to which children are willing to take risks varies greatly and can be influenced by gender, sociocultural factors, and physical abilities (Sandseter et al., 2021; Watchman & Spencer-Cavaliere, 2017).

All children approach risk differently. Some will seemingly not hesitate to partake in a risky situation; others will make conscious efforts to deliberate whether to jump in, hesitate, or eventually retreat. Factors such as sensory processing, stress, and trauma issues will also influence a child's decision to engage or not engage in risky play.

Ultimately, children choose to engage or not in risky play based on whether the reward sufficiently outweighs the perceived risk. It should be noted that children with disabilities are no different than their peers in this regard. They also benefit from risky play and should not be denied the opportunity by overly protective caregivers or designers. Studies have shown that risky play, particularly when there are opportunities to get "lost" or "disappear," is positively associated with heightened levels of physical activity, improved behavior, and better social cooperation and health (Brussoni et al., 2015; Farmer, Fitzgerald et al., 2017; Farmer, Williams et al., 2017). Inclusive[+] play spaces, in particular, should focus on providing opportunities for children to manage a broad variety of risks to meet the needs of a diverse user group. These might include opportunities to build, deconstruct, climb, and determine the best way to get back to the ground.

Social Play

Studies have shown that cooperative activities and games in the play space can effectively encourage positive social interaction (Wenger et al., 2021). Their effectiveness is attributed to positive interactions that are less frequent during other types of play (Loy & Dattilo, 2000). In fact, when play spaces lack consideration for social play, they can increase instances of social isolation and peer-group hierarchies (Massey et al., 2021). Inclusive[+] play space design provides a range of small- and large-group social opportunities for children to play that enriches their lives. These opportunities can run the gamut from two-person, fine-motor game-play spaces to larger-scale group game areas for activities such as tag, ball games, or cooperative construction. Their strategic location in the play space influences the level of social play they can impart. For example, a social play space where children make music is best located on the periphery of the play space, and a space for loose parts play should be well out of the way of swings.

Graduating Levels of Complex Play

The idea behind graduated levels of play is that the play space and its elements contain a hierarchy of motor, cognitive, and social-emotional opportunities for children to master (Lifter et al., 1993). A play space should include features that provide for a wide range of growth in skill sets and abilities, allowing everyone the chance to master the challenge and have something to move to next. One example of this concept is a sensory circuit we co-designed for an inclusive play space in Uganda (see Chapter 3 case study, Gem Village Playground). The play space is located at a residential school that serves children with multiple physical and developmental disabilities. The sensory circuit wraps around the periphery of the play space. It starts with walking-feet icons to step on, transitions to toe-walking icons, and then to jumping over lines painted on the course. In alignment with inclusive[+] design, parallel activities on the circuit provide similar experiences for children who are wheelchair users to do along the same path. The sensory circuit offers the children opportunities to master motor and cognitive skills with their peers.

Another important feature of graduated levels of complex play aligns with sensory processing, which we discuss next. Providing these play elements allows children to explore on their own terms, from low or limited sensory features, such as soft colors, smooth textures, and places to seek refuge, to more alerting features like talking tubes, highly textured materials to explore, and places to climb enables choice and autonomy.

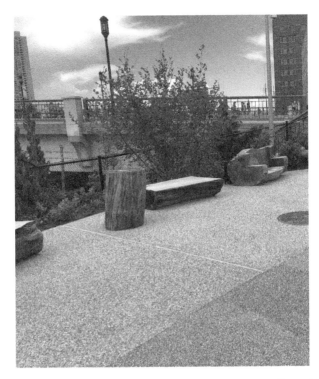

FIGURE 6.4 Variable levels of challenge with seating options. Credit- author.

When design accommodates graduated play levels, it opens up possibilities for all children to experience a sense of accomplishment and a self-esteem boost as they engage with the challenges that the play elements provide (Farmer, Fitzgerald et al., 2017; Farmer, Williams et al., 2017). There is also every likelihood that families will be more drawn to inclusive play spaces that provide many layers of challenges and options, so everyone has something fun to do (Washington et al., 2019) (see Figure 6.4).

Sensory-Focused Play

Sensory-focused play is one method children use to experience, avoid, or create the sensory input levels they personally need to develop. Most children fall into four primary groups. They may be children with (1) a high tolerance for sensory input who respond passively, (2) a high tolerance for sensory input who respond actively, (3) a low tolerance for input who respond passively, or (4) a low tolerance for input who respond actively (Dunn, 2009). See Table 6.3 for more information. Notably, all children are different; their preferences for sensory experiences vary, and those experiences may be beneficial or detrimental to their development. Their preferences often manifest in the children's behaviors and are outward expressions of their innate need to regulate their sensory needs.

TABLE 6.3 Sensory Styles

Sensory tolerance	*Response to sensory input*	
	Passive	*Active*
High	Child has a low level of awareness to the sensory input source	Child actively seeks a source for sensory input
Play example	A child in the play space is surrounded by a great deal of activity and sound but appears indifferent	A child in the play space who intentionally, repeatedly runs into stationary objects and jumps off the highest available platforms
Low	Child is sensitive to the sensory input source but does not avoid it	Child is sensitive to the sensory input source and actively avoids it
Play example	A child becomes agitated after getting dirty while playing in the sand but does not stop playing	A child senses they cannot handle getting dirty and avoids going near the sandpit

Source: Adapted from: Dunn (2009).

With a broad range of reactions to the same environmental inputs, it is imperative that play environments be carefully considered in advance to provide children in all four sensory typology groups with opportunities for positive and beneficial sensory input levels. One of the most effective methods of sensory planning is to observe the children who play, pretend, and actively recreate in nearby play spaces. Whether indoor classrooms, schoolyards, or public play spaces, these spaces can be designed with a range of sensory integrated activities that promote inclusive development and social interaction.

Strategies to help meet this objective are providing a broad diversity of play opportunities within which sensory-seeking children can find the extra inputs they need (musical instruments, varied textures, etc.), creating areas where inputs are highly focused, providing repetition for children who do not readily recognize the sensory source, creating areas with only a few simple inputs for children who are sensitive (e.g., enclosed sandboxes limit outside stimuli, do not require excessive movement, and provide a single texture), and creating spaces for retreat, where inputs are less invasive and can be avoided for children with low tolerances. With plenty of variety in the play environment, children with and without identified challenges can effectively customize their sensory experience to meet their particular needs. Christensen and Romero (2016) addressed the diverse ways children on the autism spectrum play and the unpredictability of their play: "Applying a multiple method approach appears to be the most effective way to support play behavior for children with autism spectrum disorder" (p. 129). Acknowledging that no two children have the same sensory needs and interests, this multiple-method approach benefits not just children on the autism spectrum but all children.

Intergenerational Play

This type of play encompasses strengthening the family relationship. Intergenerational family activities are shown to be most effectively accomplished through family leisure events that are "unique, shared, interactive, purposive, challenging and requiring sacrifice" (Hebblethwaite & Norris, 2011, p. 123). These opportunities can facilitate learning and teaching life skills, lessons learned, and family narratives and values. When engaged in intergenerational activities, children can gain new role models, develop more positive attitudes toward aging, thus reducing feelings of ageism, and learn from older adults (McAlister et al., 2019). Adults are also affected by engaging in intergenerational activities. They demonstrate improved physical and mental health, increased sense of belonging and meaning, and higher overall perceptions of improved quality of life (Giraudeau & Bailly, 2019). For both children and adults, intergenerational play can elicit feelings of belonging, connection, positive socialization, and being present and in the moment (Rosa Hernandez et al., 2022). Designing for intergenerational play in outdoor spaces is a win-win. It takes people outside, which is health promoting and brings children and adults together in the spirit of connection.

The benefits of social interaction between age groups result from far more than a structured formal gathering with people of multiple generations. Siyahhan et al. (2010) described it in the following way: "Productive intergenerational play, collaborative work between parent /[, grandparent,] and child . . . is characterized by exchange of expertise between the adult and the child around shared intentions" (p. 429). Davis et al.'s (2008) study focusing on the play between grandparents and their grandchildren discovered several common themes that occur during intergenerational play. These themes included:

- a desire for adults to share family history with the younger generation
- participation in activities that generate a sense of magic
- science and fun
- a generational connection through food

The ideal inclusive[+] intergenerational play environment would include diversity in play for all partners, complete with interactions and a playful atmosphere. The fundamental elements of intergenerational play revolve around a diverse and flexible palette of activities that appeal to a broad demographic. This does not imply a shotgun approach, cramming as many recreational features as possible into a space. Thoughtful inclusive[+] play space design creates spaces and features that function in versatile ways, engaging multiple generations in activities together. Activities and recreational features should:

- provide for a range of ability levels (children, adults, and older adults)
- be easily understandable with instructions or simple directions

- allow for unstructured (creative) play guided by the users (not prescribed)
- not create physical, mental, or social barriers (e.g., no segregated activities or excessive elevation changes)
- encourage activities that initiate intergenerational interaction, such as storytelling, playing board games, reading, preparing food, conversing quietly, gardening, and observing (Spence & Radunovich, 2008).

Creative Play

In some capacity, all types of play share the common feature of creativity. Creative play supports learning and social-emotional skills (Russ, 2003). Creative play helps build resilience and coping skills, particularly for children experiencing stress and trauma (Berger & Lahad, 2010), because it offers an alternative outlet to work through their struggles. Through creative play, children can also come up with creative solutions to problems. It could be how to involve a peer, who uses a wheelchair, in building a cozy hut from blocks or which natural materials enable the child to roll into the hut. It might be how to share time on the swings or dam a water runnel and then deal with the "flood" that ensues (see Figure 6.5).

We might argue that nature-focused play affords more opportunities for creativity, although manufactured play equipment can also support creativity. If we

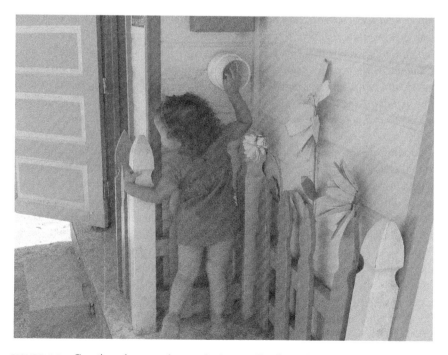

FIGURE 6.5   Creative play at a cheery playhouse. Credit- author.

dive deeper, layering inclusive⁺ play space design means that considerations must extend beyond what creative qualities a play element can provide (e.g., an interactive toy train). The design must consider how children with visible and invisible disabilities can interact with these elements in a way that, if not the same as their peers without disabilities, is very close to the same. For example, the interactive toy train we mentioned could have roll-under capacity so wheelchairs can pull up to the train engine's "controls." It could be a big enough footprint that the wheelchair can turn around with ease. This train could have color-coded elements that help children with cognitive challenges understand how the train can be activated. Some areas of the train could have limited sensory experiences (tactile, sound, visual) for children with sensory challenges; other areas would have a more alerting range of experiences. For children who need a bit of time to prepare themselves to engage with their peers and the train, a small and cozy "depot" hideaway space adjacent to the train would provide a safe refuge to observe the play and to join when and if they were ready.

Nature-Based Play

Years ago, while at a park with my nieces, I (Chad) watched a group of children from a distance as they played at a typical play space in their neighborhood. They started on the fabricated equipment, running and climbing on the structure. Not too long after we arrived, I noticed a shift in their attention: The static equipment no longer held their interest, and the lure of the adjacent unimproved land won them over. Investigating further, I found them climbing on the large limbs of a valley oak tree that hung so low they touched the ground. My nieces were searching for bugs in the decaying acorns, poking their heads through tree cavities, and arranging leaves and twigs into interesting patterns. They ended up spending most of their time in that lot and did not return to the formal play space that day. This experience is a prime example of the value that nature can play in the process of play.

Modern design philosophies now embrace incorporating plant life and other natural elements into play areas. At the core of this shift in approach is the concept that nature is intrinsically dynamic and everchanging. Adding these features to play spaces introduces limitless variety, change, and opportunities for creativity. Natural elements can be incorporated into play areas in ways that reflect safety regulations, risk-management programs, and maintenance requirements.

First and foremost, nature is always changing, providing children with renewable supplies of play materials, sensory experiences, and creeping critters. In essence, play areas integrated with natural elements are different and afford new experiences each time a child visits. Logically, this type of play area retains its novelty over time, encouraging more frequent visits. According to R. C. Moore et al. (2009), "Diverse [natural] play settings meet individual needs according to stages of development, learning styles, personality types, friendship patterns and culture" (p. 5). These types of spaces endure the test of time as desirable destinations for children and their caregivers. Research also showed that children find symbolism in nature that directly correlates with creative play (Johnson, 2009).

Additionally, including natural elements provides an educational experience that nurtures hands-on learning and exploration, which seldom exists in traditional play spaces, particularly those with an inclusive focus. Exploration is also a fundamental form of play, an innate draw to natural settings, and is crucial to helping a child understand the surrounding landscape. Natural features, such as inert materials, landforms, seed pods, flowers, grasses, trees, insects, and other wildlife, are all curious specimens worthy of childlike exploration and investigation (see Figure 6.6).

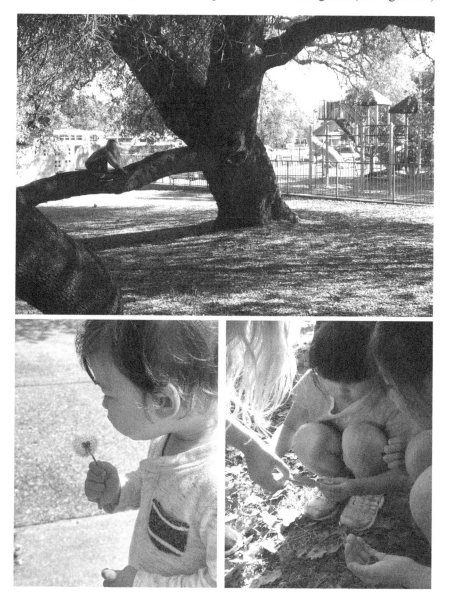

FIGURE 6.6   Engaging in spontaneous gross and fine motor sensory-based nature play. Credit- author and Ben Atchison.

Trauma-Responsive Play

Children who have experienced, or are experiencing, trauma in their lives need opportunities to play; it is an essential part of what they need to grow and develop. Trauma in childhood is often referred to as *adverse childhood experiences* (ACEs). These experiences can change a child's brain structure and development and affect how they respond to stress. Some reasons children develop ACEs include maternal depression, physical and emotional neglect, caregiver divorce, mental illness, incarceration, being unhoused, experiencing or witnessing domestic violence, caregiver substance abuse, or emotional or sexual abuse. The more ACEs a child has, the more likely they are to be long-term and negatively impacted, as manifested in the ways they interact with others, feel about themselves (Centers for Disease Control and Prevention, 2021; Harvard Center on the Developing Child, 2023), learn, and move their bodies. Play allows children to experience a whole new world, and inclusive[+] play space design is well suited to be trauma responsive, which we briefly explore in Chapter 7, "Design Guidelines."

It is beyond the scope of this book to provide detailed information about or guidelines for trauma-responsive design for outdoor play spaces. However, all designers can be aware of some basic ideas to support children with trauma histories. These ideas we developed are applicable to any outdoor play space, whether or not intended to be inclusive.

- Provide a variety of sensory experiences that nourish all eight sensory systems, taking care to think about offering alerting and calming options.
- Choice is important! Select options for play experiences from simple to complex.
- Create cozy and snug spaces, whether inside the play space or along the periphery, that provide a sense of safety and comfort for children who need to self-regulate.
- Natural and vegetative materials are also important to consider. Be aware of textures and colors and select carefully to provide a range of sensory experiences like smelling, touching, hearing, and seeing.
- Consider consistency and repetition in your design because both tend to be grounding and calming. Repetition and consistency could come in the form of an easily understandable hierarchy of color choices, signage, and pathway shapes and sizes. This is not to suggest avoiding a bit of mystery and novelty— just minimize it in favor of predictability.

Final Thoughts

A long-standing and interesting history of inclusive play space design spans federal legislation and code, the design community, education, and therapy research. It represents a giant step forward from accessible design focused on mobility issues. Inclusive[+] play space design takes inclusive design to a more individual, child-centered level by viewing the physical environment as just one part of the process. Planning for social considerations deepens the design process. Even more so, physical and social design must be informed by equity, so all children have opportunities to do what they need to do—play. Play is, for children, a key to healthy development. Design can facilitate play in the best ways possible.

BOX 6.1   CASE STUDY: ADDY GRACE PLAYGROUND (FIGURES 6.7–6.9)

Project Information:

Description:

Name
Addy Grace Playground
Designer
Sparks at Play and
Landscape Structures,
Inc.
Location
Daleville, VA
Size
1,010 m² or 0.25 acre
Year Built
2019
Age Group
2–5 years, 5–12 years

The champions for this play space were Addy Grace's parents, who wanted to have an enriching play experience for both of their children. The design is based on an agricultural theme to align with the rural setting within which it was built. The design was set up to encourage interactions between Addy Grace, who uses a reclined wheelchair, and her brother, who is ambulatory. Hence, the planning and design revolved around providing similar and shared experiences at each event. This concept led to having social play at varying levels. Although the play area is small, it is large in play value and play diversity. The space allows and features many play experiences beyond the play structures themselves. The community was highly engaged with the project and its fundraising.

Website:

• http://addygracefoundation.com/help-us-build-the-farm/

Traditional Inclusive Features	Inclusive+ Features
• Accessible path of travel • Accessible structures • Accessible spinners • PIP rubber surfacing • Accessible slides • Accessible climbers • Completely fenced perimeter for safety	• Plenty of ground-accessible play features reduces the physical effort necessary to navigate the play space • Double-wide paths provide comfortable and shared access to high-interest play features, like the tractor and rocking trailer • Double-wide slides encourage social interaction and play • Built adjacent to the YMCA building for easy access to comfort facilities and complimentary indoor activities • Dramatic play elements, such as the produce stations, encourage peer and intergenerational social interaction • The agricultural theme is familiar, relatable, and comfortable for children living in the region

(Continued)

(Continued)

Traditional Inclusive Features	Inclusive+ Features
• Transition stations are located nearby the bottom of slide exit chutes	• Themed zones and path hierarchy for easy understanding of the play opportunities • Creative and dramatic play themed seek-and-find games

Remarks:

Several features of the Addy Grace play space align with the concepts we identify as being inclusive+, such as its sociogeographical focus and double-wide paths. However, overall, we feel it better represents a typical approach to inclusive design. This mighty play area packs a lot of activity into a limited space. It also does a wonderful job of integrating community relevance in a way that is familiar, relatable, and comforting for the users. A very clever example of this is the farm direction signage, which names all the local farms that contributed to the project. Almost everyone in the community can relate to these farms, and the playful signage provides a sense of grounding and belonging to where they are in the world and their community. Myriad small details around and hidden within the play space bolster the agricultural theme and make a creative and enriching exploratory experience. Another well-integrated concept is that of diverse play opportunities. In addition to the sociogeographical-(agriculture)-themed play structure with climbers, panels, and slides, the remainder of the play area is filled with other challenges. They include multiple types of spinners, different types of rocking elements, swings, an adapted zipline, seek-and-find games, strategic photo opportunities, a multitude of sensory talk tubes, and a roller table for tactile, proprioceptive, and vestibular input. This diversity in play features allows and encourages graduating levels of mastery as children learn and grow.

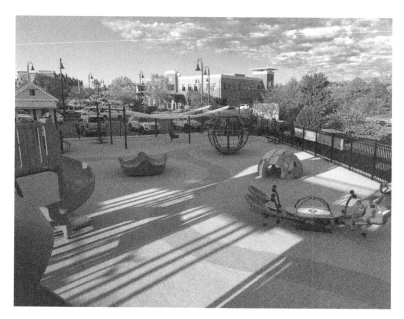

FIGURE 6.7   Play zones are clearly delineated with color changes in poured in place paving. Credit- Sparks at Play.

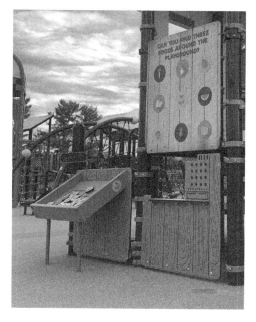

FIGURE 6.8   Universally accessible play stations welcome sitting and standing visitors. Credit- Sparks at Play.

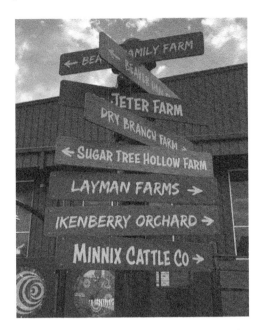

FIGURE 6.9   Signs link the play space to the community at large. Photo by Sparks at Play.

BOX 6.2 CENTENNIAL PARK (FIGURES 6.10–6.12)

Project Information: **Description:**

Name
Centennial Park
Designer
O'Dell Engineering

Location
Madera, CA
Size
1,115 m² or 0.28 acre
Year Built
2016
Age Group(s)
2–5 years, 5–12 years

With an identified strong community need for a socially inclusive play space, the city of Madera, California, and its citizens worked together to create an accessible, unique, and engaging recreational opportunity. Funded through a low-income incentive program, the project included renovations to the existing Centennial Park adjacent to the John W. Wells Youth Center. Improvements include a socially inclusive play space, ADA-access retrofits, new site lighting, irrigation retrofits, accessible restrooms, and picnic facilities.

Being a socially inclusive play space, a wide variety of activities and exciting aesthetics in the space are key. The centerpiece is a custom play structure accessed via sloped pathways to ensure equitable use. The theme of the park is a road trip through California. Custom elements found in the play space include a wave path, giving children opportunities to challenge their balance skills in a fun way. There is also a play cabin for refuge and self-regulation. Custom sculptural elements depicting oversized California poppies provide color and wayfinding cues. The plants in the surrounding landscape also play into this theme: hardy manzanita plants reference the Sierra Mountain range landscape, and dwarf olive plants acknowledge their agricultural significance in the California Central Valley. Other plant species were specifically chosen for their flowers, seed pods, cones, and other parts that are useful in loose-parts play.

Website:

- https://www.madera.gov/home/departments/parks-community-services/parks-trails/

Traditional Inclusive Features	Inclusive⁺ Features
• Accessible path of travel • Accessible structure • Accessible swings • PIP rubber surfacing	• Having no ramps significantly reduced the physical effort to navigate the play space • Nature-based theme to enhance exploratory play options • Double-wide roller slide to encourage social play
• Accessible slides • Completely fenced perimeter for safety	• Multiple cozy spaces for self-regulation and restoration • Multisensory integrated trail stops with musical equipment • Accessible gender-neutral restroom • Integrated landscape/natural elements to encourage loose-parts play • Integrated grade changes, such as an undulating path that provides movement challenges • Overarching play approach focused on social-emotional connections and learning • Integrated companion seating benches and tables for comfort and socialization • Play-related dramatic art features encourages imaginative play and interaction • Integrated and natural shade options to help with temperature and internal regulation

(Continued)

(Continued)

Remarks:

This project is a good example of how, with limited budget and grant restrictions, a play space can be creatively designed to maximize inclusive⁺ play value while remaining practical. The budget did not allow complete coverage of the play space with a unitary play surface, so the play space features were carefully sited and provided with access, leaving some duplicate features and use areas with loose-fill surfacing. This is a reasonable compromise between budget and the need for physical access. The thematic elements are well placed to foster dramatic play in the 2- to 5-year-old area. Multiple cozy spaces on either end of the play space are well situated to allow children the option to self-regulate away from busy play, while still providing visual access and proximity to the action. Walkways are gently sloped to allow reaching higher platforms without significant expenditure of effort. They lead to a central spine between the younger and older children's areas. For such a small space, this play space offers abundant activities and diverse play opportunities for family engagement.

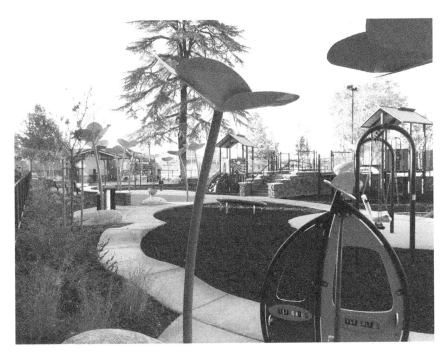

FIGURE 6.10 A balance of sensory rich graded challenges welcome all children to play together. Credit- author.

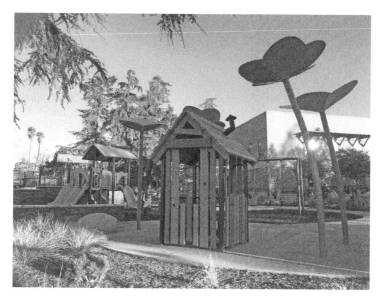

FIGURE 6.11   Cozy spaces located outside the main play areas allow children to seek prospect and refuge when overwhelmed or engage in creative and dramatic play. Credit- author.

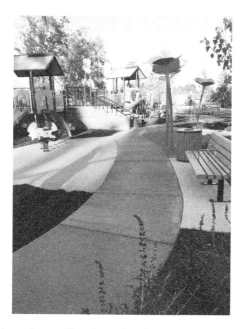

FIGURE 6.12   If budgets do not allow for entire play area to have poured in place paving an alternative is a highly contrasting colored poured in place pad area around play elements with easy access from major routes of travel. Credit- author.

References

Americans with Disabilities Act of 1990, 42 U.S.C. § 121010 *et seq.* (1990). https://www.ada.gove/pubs/adastatute08.htm

Architectural and Transportation Barriers Compliance Board. (2000). *Americans with Disabilities Act (ADA) accessibility guidelines for buildings and facilities: Play areas; final rule.* https://www.govinfo.gov/content/pkg/FR-2000-10-18/pdf/00-26466.pdf#page=2

Aslaksen, F., Bergh, S., Bringa, O. R., & Heggem, E. K. (1997). *The gap model of disability.* [Infographic]. The Norwegian State Council on Disability. https://www.independentliving.org/docs1/nscd1997.html

Berger, R., & Lahad, M. (2010). A safe place: Ways in which nature, play and creativity can help children cope with stress and crisis; establishing the kindergarten as a safe haven where children can develop resiliency. *Early Child Development and Care, 180*(7), 889–900. https://doi.org/10.1080/03004430802525013

Brown, D. M., Ross, T., Leo, J., Buliung, R. N., Shirazipour, C. H., Latimer-Cheung, A. E., & Arbour-Nicitopoulos, K. P. (2021). A scoping review of evidence-informed recommendations for designing inclusive playgrounds. *Frontiers in Rehabilitation Sciences, 2*, Article 664595. https://doi.org/10.3389/fresc.2021.664595

Brussoni, M., Olsen, L. L., Pike, I., & Sleet, D. A. (2012). Risky play and children's safety: Balancing priorities for optimal child development. *International Journal of Environmental Research and Public Health, 9*(9), 3134–3148. https://doi.org/10.3390/ijerph9093134

Brussoni, M., Gibbons, R., Gray, C., Ishikawa, T., Sandseter, E. B. H., Bienenstock, A., Chabot, G., Fuselli, P., Herrington, S., Janssen, I., Pickett, W., Power, M., Stanger, N., Sampson, M., & Tremblay, M. S. (2015). What is the relationship between risky outdoor play and health in children? A systematic review. *International Journal of Environmental Research and Public Health, 12*(6), 6423–6454. https://doi.org/10.3390/ijerph120606423

Commission for Architecture and the Built Environment. (2006). *The principles of inclusive design. (They include you).* CABE. https://www.designcouncil.org.uk/fileadmin/uploads/dc/Documents/the-principles-of-inclusive-design.pdf

Centers for Disease Control and Prevention. (2021). *Adverse childhood experiences (ACES): Preventing early trauma to improve adult health.* https://www.cdc.gov/vitalsigns/aces/index.html

Christensen, K. M., & Jeon, T. K. (2006). Creating inclusive outdoor play environments: Designing for ability rather than disability. *Journal of Eyewitness in Special Education, 910*, 48–55.

Christensen, K., & Romero, L. P. R. (2016). Creating outdoor play environments to support social interactions of children with autism spectrum disorder: A scoping study. *Landscape Research Record, 5*, 128–140.

Coates, J. K., & Pimlott-Wilson, H. (2019). Learning while playing: Children's forest school experiences in the UK. *British Educational Research Journal, 45*(1), 21–40. https://doi.org/10.1002/berj.3491

Davis, H., Vetere, F., Francis, P., Gibbs, M., & Howard, S. (2008). "I wish we could get together": Exploring intergenerational play across a distance via a "Magic Box." *Journal of Intergenerational Relationships, 6*(2), 191–210. https://doi.org/10.1080/15350770801955321

Dunn, W. (2009). *Living sensationally: Understanding your senses.* Jessica Kinglsey.

Farmer, V. L., Fitzgerald, R. P., Williams, S. M., Mann, J. I., Schofield, G., McPhee, J. C., & Taylor, R. W. (2017). What did schools experience from participating in a randomised controlled study (PLAY) that prioritised risk and challenge in active play for children while at school? *Journal of Adventure Education and Outdoor Learning, 17*(3), 239–257. https://doi.org/10.1080/14729679.2017.1286993

Farmer, V. L., Williams, S. M., Mann, J. I., Schofield, G., McPhee, J. C., & Taylor, R. W. (2017). The effect of increasing risk and challenge in the school playground on physical activity and weight in children: A cluster randomised controlled trial (PLAY). *International Journal of Obesity, 41*(5), 793–800. https://doi.org/10.1038/ijo.2017.41

Giraudeau, C., & Bailly, N. (2019). Intergenerational programs: What can school-age children and older people expect from them? A systematic review. *European Journal of Ageing, 16*, 363–376. https://doi.org/10.1007/s10433-018-00497-4

Gleave, J. (2008). *Risk and play: A literature review*. PlayDay. https://www.springzaad.nl/wp-content/uploads/2020/04/risk_and_play-a_literature_review.pdf

Goodley, D., & Runswick-Cole, K. (2010). Emancipating play: Dis/abled children, development and deconstruction. *Disability & Society, 25*(4), 499–512. https://doi.org/10.1080/09687591003755914

Graham, N. E., Truman, J., & Holgate, H. (2015). Parents' understanding of play for children with cerebral palsy. *American Journal of Occupational Therapy, 69*(3), 6903220050p1–6903220050p9. https://doi.org/10.5014/ajot.2015.015263

Gray, P. (2020). Risky play: Why children love and need it. In J. Loebach, S. Little, A. Cox, & P. Eubanks Owens (Eds.), *The Routledge handbook of designing public spaces for young people* (pp. 39–51). Routledge.

Harvard Center on the Developing Child. (2023). *ACEs and toxic stress: Frequently asked questions*. https://developingchild.harvard.edu/resources/aces-and-toxic-stress-frequently-asked-questions/

Hazlehurst, M. F., Muqueeth, S., Wolf, K. L., Simmons, C., Kroshus, E., & Tandon, P. S. (2022). Park access and mental health among parents and children during the COVID-19 pandemic. *BMC Public Health, 22*(1). https://doi.org/10.1186/s12889-022-13148-2

Hebblethwaite, S., & Norris, J. (2011). Expressions of generativity through family leisure: Experiences of grandparents and adult grandchildren. *Family Relations, 60*, 121–133. https://doi.org/10.1111/j.1741-3729.2010.00637.x

Individuals with Disabilities Education Act, 20 U.S.C. § 1400. (2004). https://sites.ed.gov/idea/statute-chapter-33/subchapter-i/1400

Institute for Human Centered Design. (n.d.). *What is universal design . . . inclusive design . . . design-for-all?* https://ihcd-api.s3.amazonaws.com/s3fs-public/file+downloads/Inclusive+Design+Cheat+Sheet+6+18.pdf

Johnson, J. M. (2009). *Design for learning: Values, qualities, and processes of enriching school landscapes*. American Society of Landscape Architects.

Johnstone, A., Martin, A., Cordovil, R., Fjørtoft, I., Iivonen, S., Jidovtseff, B., Lopes, F., Reilly, J. J., Thomson, H., Wells, V., & McCrorie, P. (2022). Nature-based early childhood education and children's social, emotional and cognitive development: A mixed-methods systematic review. *International Journal of Environmental Research and Public Health, 19*(10), 5967. https://doi.org/10.3390/ijerph19105967

Kelly, R., & Mutebi, N. (2023). *Invisible disabilities in education and employment* [POST-note 689]. UK Parliament Post. https://researchbriefings.files.parliament.uk/documents/POST-PN-0689/POST-PN-0689.pdf

LaPiere, R., & Dion, L. (2022). Using nature to create safety for medical trauma integration. In J. A. Courtney, J. L. Langley, L. L. Wonders, R. Heiko, & R. LaPiere (Eds.), *Nature-based play and expressive therapies: Interventions for working with children, teens, and families* (pp. 83–97). Routledge.

Lifter, K., Sulzer-Azaroff, B., Anderson, S. R., & Cowdery, G. E. (1993). Teaching play activities to preschool children with disabilities: The importance of developmental considerations. *Journal of Early Intervention, 17*(2), 139–159. https://doi.org/10.1177/105381519301700206

Loy, D. P., & Dattilo, J. (2000). Effects of different play structures on social interactions between a boy with Asperger's syndrome and his peers. *Therapeutic Recreation Journal, 34*(3), 190–210.

Lynch, H., Moore, A., Edwards, C., & Horgan, L. (2020). Advancing play participation for all: The challenge of addressing play diversity and inclusion in community parks and playgrounds. *British Journal of Occupational Therapy, 83*(2), 107–117. https://doi.org/10.1177/0308022619881

Massey, W. V., Perez, D., Neilson, L., Thalken, J., & Szarabajko, A. (2021). Observations from the playground: Common problems and potential solutions for school-based recess. *Health Education Journal, 80*(3), 313–326. https://doi.org/10.1177/00178969209733190.

Mather, J. (1981). *Learning can be child's play*. Abington Press.

McAlister, J., Briner, E. L., & Maggi, S. (2019). Intergenerational programs in early childhood education: An innovative approach that highlights inclusion and engagement with older adults. *Journal of Intergenerational Relationships, 17*(4), 505–522. https://doi.org/10.1080/15350770.2019.1618777

Moore, A., Lynch, H., & Boyle, B. (2022). Can universal design support outdoor play, social participation, and inclusion in public playgrounds? A scoping review. *Disability and Rehabilitation, 44*(13), 3304–3325. https://doi.org/10.1080/09638288.2020.1858353

Moore, R. C., Cosco, N., Sherk, J., Bieber, B., Varela, S., Gurina, N., & Murphy, J. (2009). *Creating & retrofitting play environments: Best practice guidelines*. Playcore, Inc. and Natural Learning Initiative, College of Design, NC State University. https://www.play-core.com/programs/naturegrounds

Morgan, P. (2020, March 20). Invisible disabilities: Break down the barriers. *Forbes*. https://www.forbes.com/sites/paulamorgan/2020/03/20/invisible-disabilities-break-down-the-barriers/?sh=6763cfddfa50

Murniyati, B., & Wardhani, J. D. (2023). Economic token techniques as an effort to increase the independence of children aged 4–5 Years. *Early Childhood Research Journal, 5*(2), 29–43. https://doi.org/10.23917/ecrj.v5i2.20834

Mygind, L., Kjeldsted, E., Hartmeyer, R., Mygind, E., Bølling, M., & Bentsen, P. (2019). Mental, physical and social health benefits of immersive nature-experience for children and adolescents: A systematic review and quality assessment of the evidence. *Health & Place, 58*, Article 102136. https://doi.org/10.1016/j.healthplace.2019.05.014

NC State University Center for Universal Design. (1997). *The principles of universal design*. https://projects.ncsu.edu/ncsu/design/cud/about_ud/udprinciplestext.htm

Obee, P., Sandseter, E. B. H., Gerlach, A., & Harper, N. J. (2021). Lessons learned from Norway on risky play in early childhood education and care (ECEC). *Early Childhood Education Journal, 49*, 99–109. https://doi.org/10.1007/s10643-020-01044-6

Owen, C., McCann, D., Rayner, C., & Wells, J. (2017). Design across the spectrum: Enhancing inclusion for children on the autism spectrum in the playground. In D. Barron & K. Seeman (Eds.), *Proceedings of the Fourth International Conference on Design4Health 2017* (pp. 169–176). Sheffield Hallam University and Swinburne University of Technology.

Patrick, V. M., & Hollenbeck, C. R. (2021). Designing for all: Consumer response to inclusive design. *Journal of Consumer Psychology, 31*(2), 360–381. https://doi.org/10.1002/jcpy.1225

Persson, H., Åhman, H., Yngling, A. A., & Gulliksen, J. (2015). Universal design, inclusive design, accessible design, design for all: Different concepts—one goal? On the concept of accessibility—historical, methodological and philosophical aspects. *Universal Access in the Information Society, 14*(4), 505–526. https://doi.org/10.1007/s10209-014-0358-z

Prellwitz, M., & Skär, L. (2007). Usability of playgrounds for children with different abilities. *Occupational Therapy International, 14*, 44–55. https://doi.org/10.1002/oti.230

Radzi, N. A. M., Ismail, K., & Ab Wahab, L. (2020). Ergonomics concept in inclusive public playground targeting on children with disabilities. *Environment-Behaviour Proceedings Journal, 5*(15), 3–9. https://doi.org/10.21834/ebpj.v5i15.2499

Rehabilitation Act, 29 U.S.C. § 540 *et seq.* (1973). https://www.govinfo.gov/app/details/CFR-2002-title28-vol1/CFR-2002-title28-vol1-

Right to Play. (2022). *History of boundless playgrounds.* http://righttoplay.org/about-us/boundless-playgrounds/

Rosa Hernandez, G. B., Murray, C. M., & Stanley, M. (2022). An intergenerational playgroup in an Australian residential aged-care setting: A qualitative case study. *Health & Social Care in the Community, 30*(2), 488–497. https://doi.org/10.1111/hsc.13149

Russ, S. W. (2003). Play and creativity: Developmental issues. *Scandinavian Journal of Educational Research, 47*(3), 291–303. https://doi.org/10.1080/00313830308594

Sandseter, E. B. H. (2007). Categorising risky play: How can we identify risk-taking in children's play? *European Early Childhood Education Research Journal, 15*(2), 237–252. https://doi.org/10.1080/13502930701321733

Sandseter, E. B. H. (2009). Affordances for risky play in preschool: The importance of features in the play environment. *Early Childhood Education Journal, 36*, 439–446. https://doi.org/10.1007/s10643-009-0307-2

Sandseter, E. B. H., Kleppe, R., & Sando, O. J. (2021). The prevalence of risky play in young children's indoor and outdoor free play. *Early Childhood Education Journal, 49*, 303–312. https://doi.org/10.1007/s10643-020-01074-0

Siyahhan, S., Barab, S. A., & Downton, M. P. (2010). Using activity theory to understand intergenerational play: The case of Family Quest. *International Journal of Computer-Supported Collaborative Learning, 5*, 415–432. https://doi.org/10.1007/s11412-010-9097-1

Smith, K. E., & Pollak, S. D. (2020). Early life stress and development: Potential mechanisms for adverse outcomes. *Journal of Neurodevelopmental Disorders, 12*, 1–15. https://doi.org/10.1186/s11689-020-09337-y

Spence, L., & Radunovich, H. L. (2008). *Developing intergenerational relationships.* University of Florida IFAS Extension, FCS2282 [Course]. https://doi.org/10.32473/edis-fy1007-2007

Stanton-Chapman, T. L., & Schmidt, E. L. (2017). Creating an inclusive playground for children of all abilities: West Fork Playground in Cincinnati, Ohio. *Children, Youth and Environments, 27*(3), 124–137. https://doi.org/10.7721/chilyoutenvi.27.3.0124

Stenman, K., Christofferson, J., Alderfer, M. A., Pierce, J., Kelly, C., Schifano, E., Klaff, S., Sciolla, J., Deatrick, J., & Kazak, A. E. (2019). Integrating play in trauma-informed care: Multidisciplinary pediatric healthcare provider perspectives. *Psychological Services, 16*(1), 7–15. https://doi.org/10.1037/ser0000294

Sunarty, K., & Dirawan Darma, G. (2015). Development parenting model to increase the independence of children. *International Education Studies, 8*(10), 107–113. https://doi.org/10.5539/ies.v8n10p107

Tai, L. (2022). *Letting play bloom: Designing nature-based risky play for children.* Temple University Press.

UNICEF. (2012). *Convention on the rights of the child*. https://www.unicef.org/child-rights-convention/convention-text#

UNICEF. (2021, November 9). *Nearly 240 million children with disabilities around the world, UNICEF's most comprehensive statistical analysis finds* [Press release]. https://www.unicef.org/press-releases/nearly-240-million-children-disabilities-around-world-unicefs-most-comprehensive

U.S. Census Bureau. (2021). *Childhood disability in the United States: 2019*. https://www.census.gov/library/publications/2021/acs/acsbr-006.html

U.S. Department of Agriculture. (2012). *Accessibility guidebook for outdoor recreation and trails*. https://www.fs.usda.gov/sites/default/files/Accessibility-Guide-Book.pdf

U.S. Department of Justice (2010). *2010 ADA Standards for accessible design*. https://www.ada.gov/law-and-regs/design-standards/2010-stds/

Van Melik, R., & Althuizen, N. (2022). Inclusive play policies: Disabled children and their access to Dutch playgrounds. *Journal of Economic and Human Geography, 113*(2), 117–130. https://doi.org/10.1111/tesg.12457

Washington, T. L., Flanders Cushing, D., Mackenzie, J., Buys, L., & Trost, S. (2019). Fostering social sustainability through intergenerational engagement in Australian neighborhood parks. *Sustainability, 11*(16), Article 4435. https://doi.org/10.3390/su11164435

Watchman, T., & Spencer-Cavaliere, N. (2017). Times have changed: Parent perspectives on children's free play and sport. *Psychology of Sport and Exercise, 32*, 102–112. https://doi.org/10.1016/j.psychsport.2017.06.008

Wenger, I., Schulze, C., Lundström, U., & Prellwitz, M. (2021). Children's perceptions of playing on inclusive playgrounds: A qualitative study. *Scandinavian Journal of Occupational Therapy, 28*(2), 136–146. https://doi.org/10.1080/11038128.2020.1810768

7

DESIGN GUIDELINES

Introduction

Throughout the world and in every culture, children play. For some children, play does not come naturally due to personal factors, such as physical, social-emotional, or cognitive challenges. For others, sociogeographic and demographic environmental barriers, such as the lack of access to play spaces or the play environment itself, limit play. As advocates for all children's right to play, we take good design to a higher level with inclusive[+] play space design guidelines. These are a road map to creating a play environment that welcomes all children and their caregivers to be part of what should be the most natural part of childhood—play. In this chapter, we explore strategies for designing inclusive[+] play spaces. We invite you to take this information and build onto our strategies to create your most compassionate and impactful inclusive[+] play space where all children can and do thrive.

Play Space Location Selection

A centralized, evidence-supported information repository associated with where inclusive play spaces have been or are being constructed throughout the world is not to be found. In 2013, an app called "Playgrounds for Everyone" was launched to invite the public to help identify accessible play spaces in the United States (National Public Radio, 2013). Although the app is no longer live and had focused on accessibility versus inclusion, it represented the increasing interest in providing children with disabilities and their families "go-to" information for places to play. The needle has not moved much further in the decade between launching that app and writing this book. The mainstream literature contains no evidence-based "go-to" resources providing information about the locations of inclusive play spaces.

DOI: 10.4324/9781003193890-7

An extensive literature search of peer-reviewed studies identified only one research article. This study reported that about 460 playgrounds (70%) in Hong Kong were identified as inclusive, yet less than 5% included inclusive amenities (Siu et al., 2017). This is a call to action!

Further, there is limited agreement and research on what an inclusive play space is or what the policies associated with their design should be (Van Melik & Althuizen, 2022). This brings us to our next point: What features and elements found in play spaces make them inclusive? A recent and promising systematic review of the literature on inclusive play space design distilled 13 recommendations into five broad categories important for inclusive play space design: entry points, surfacing and paths, features to foster inclusive play, staffing/supervision, and the design process (Brown et al., 2021, pp. 6–9). This lack of research about what it means to be an inclusive play space has led to difficulty in developing an accurate information repository from which to identify inclusive play spaces. It has also limited the potential to research how these spaces influence children's health and development.

Trends

In learning about inclusive play spaces and how we apply this understanding to the design work we do, we noticed some trends in inclusive spaces. Although not scientific or evidence-based, we observed that these trends tend to reflect sociodemographic and sociogeographic patterns. For instance, many inclusive play space projects are funded through community and philanthropic-based fundraising. Resources such as Kaboom, play equipment manufacturers, and other outdoor-play-focused organizations often devote a section of their websites to grant resources funding inclusive play space projects.

Further, many inclusive play space projects are built in areas with more expendable income and where fundraising is more feasible. In areas lacking community interest and a champion to organize a group, the process of bringing an inclusive play space project to the neighborhood is daunting. In underrepresented communities, other needs—such as basic subsistence—may take higher priorities than having a play space.

When inclusive play space site selections are under consideration, decisions are often made based on available parkland, parking access, existing parks needing renovation, or proximity to families or businesses that donate to the cause. Not often enough do the community's or region's sociocultural demographics influence the location of a new play space. Often, however, the communities that most need play spaces have children living in underrepresented or marginalized communities and at high risk for global developmental delays (Gil et al., 2020; Smythe et al., 2021).

On top of being socioeconomically disadvantaged, children living in marginalized communities or neighborhoods may be doubly disadvantaged—they may have identified disabilities or conditions (or may exhibit characteristics of disabilities or conditions not yet diagnosed) and are not receiving needed support. Hence, the double disadvantage factor exacerbates an already-at-risk situation for healthy childhood development. A thoughtful review of the community's demographics and collaboration with local nonprofits and other social service agencies serving underrepresented populations is imperative. Doing so will help identify areas where populations in need are greatest and inclusive play spaces could be most impactful.

Inclusive play space projects tend to become destination locations because so many families need them. The adage "If you build it, they will come" applies in this circumstance. Families who need an inclusive play space and have the ability and/or means to get there will go. However, some will not have the capability or means to reach an inclusive play space. Playing outdoors is precious, and everyone needs the opportunity to do so. More so, they need to do so without it being a burden to get to.

Some of these trends, albeit anecdotal in nature, raise concerns from an environmental justice perspective. We see a possible connection between the presence and quality of inclusive play spaces in higher income areas and better health for those who use them—as well as poorer health outcomes for persons with disabilities who lack access to outdoor play spaces, inclusive or not (Jenkins et al., 2015). The term *equigenesis* refers to places that reduce health inequities (Mitchell et al., 2014). These spaces "act to disrupt the usual conversion of socioeconomic adversity to a greater risk of poor health . . . [and] may include recreational/green areas" (Mitchell et al., 2015, p. 83). To date, the research that looked at disparities in geographical location and poorer health outcomes has been conducted primarily on green spaces. Although it highlights the benefits of access to green space and not specifically play spaces, equigenics seems well suited to tying childhood activities in green spaces to outdoor play spaces. In a 2020 interview, Dr. Cathy Jordan linked equigenesis with children and nature.

> The term is used in our sector to refer to when nature benefits children negatively impacted by economic disadvantage even more than it benefits children from more advantaged backgrounds. So, although nature might be good for all children, it's especially good for those who might be at risk for poorer health, mental health, social or educational outcomes as a result of factors associated with limited financial resources. The implication is that equitable access to nature could, for example, help close educational achievement gaps or reduce health disparities.
>
> *(Children and Nature Network, 2020, para. 1)*

Considerations

When planning an inclusive[+] play project to provide the most benefit possible, think about equigenesis. Consider local community demographics, sociogeographic economics, health, age, and many other factors. Research each factor thoroughly and weigh their impact on children and their families before selecting any final site. There are many other factors to consider when looking for the best play space site. For renovations or completely new builds, the following paragraphs contain a few thoughts to consider.

Site Selection

Most municipalities have a park hierarchy in their parks master plans or general plans. Typically, these plans note within the hierarchies what types of allowed amenities apply to each park category. Community parks (often 5 acres and larger) have the most potential for inclusive play space renovations because they allow or already have restrooms and parking. Many municipalities will not allow on-site parking or restrooms in smaller parks.

Look for parks with existing safety features, like lighting, cameras, and fencing already installed. Although these safety features can often be installed with the play space, time and money can be saved if this infrastructure is already in place. Note that existing grade changes (not completely flat) can benefit site work, so play equipment ramps are less needed.

Look for parks and areas where play spaces are below the per capita threshold requirements (typically found in a city's general plans, often visioning documents identifying a city's objectives, principles, policies, and standards). An industry standard in the United States is that parks be within walking distance (0.25–0.50 miles) from any home. Look for areas where this may not be the case or where a park within that distance lacks amenities for children and families.

Access

After identifying potential locations for an inclusive play space, review the area around the site to determine whether there are pedestrian-friendly walkways to the park from the surrounding neighborhoods. Follow up this area survey by determining whether the walkways and crosswalks are accessible. If they are not, consider looking elsewhere for a site: Not only must the play space itself be inclusive, but—at a minimum—an accessible route to get there is necessary. Identify whether there is access to public transportation at the proposed play space location.

Many families with disabilities make frequent trips to health care facilities for treatments and check-ups. Would available parks or locations near these facilities be well suited for an inclusive play space?

Funding

Determine whether the park is in an area that would be compatible/eligible within potential local, state, and federal grant guidelines. Securing funding can be a significant challenge when there is a conflict with eligibility. Examples of conditions to be aware of in typical grant requirements include the following restrictions:

- Matching fund requirements
- Grant deadline windows for proposals and construction
- Eligible applicants (municipalities, joint powers authorities, nonprofit organizations, etc.)
- Project location must be in a park-deficient or economically disadvantaged area
- Designation and commitment that the area be placed into permanent park use
- The park has not received previous grant funds from the same source
- A public input process may need to be completed (we highly recommend facilitating this in any project, no matter the grant guidelines)

The Land and Water Conservation Fund is a good resource program to learn about common funding requirements in the United States. Their website (https://lwcfcoalition.org/state-and-local-assistance) provides background, program requirements, and prerequisites typical of many grant programs (https://lwcfcoalition.org/state-and-local-assistance). State programs administer these funds; therefore, many US states model their grants after applicable federal programs. A comprehensive example of this is the California State Parks Application Guide for Land and Water Conservation Grants (State of California Natural Resources Agency, 2023).

Design Strategies

Be intentional and user-focused with your design process. Not every inclusive+ play space will or should be the same because each play space environment and site condition varies. In addition, every user group is different, such that the site and users' needs collectively require a unique design approach. Knowing as much as possible about the play space type, users, site managers, and supervisors before beginning design is also critical to help you understand how the space will be maintained. For example, this information allows planning for visitors who rely on service animals by providing amenities such as water fountains with pet bowls, waste stations, and pet relief zones. Tuning into the considerations associated with the three common play space types—outdoor, public, and semipublic—can help you get off on the right foot as you begin designing an inclusive+ play space.

Community and Public Spaces

Play spaces that are entirely open to the public can be a challenge. Typically, they have no mechanisms in place for continuous, 24-hour observation or oversight of public places. Any design approach for public spaces needs to include forethought around several considerations, such as equipment maintenance, potential for vandalism, and exposure to the elements.

Recognize that public amenities must be robust and built for rigorous, repetitive, and frequent use. One of the most discouraging scenarios is expending tremendous energy to install a play space that becomes an instant hit and is loved by the community—so much that it falls into disrepair in just a short time. This frequently happens as budgets are cut. Accordingly, strong "bulletproof" equipment and materials should be substituted for inferior products.

No product on the market will be completely immune to intense use that occurs in public places, but smart decisions can help prolong the need for replacements. Examples include avoiding cheaply built play equipment that bends, dents, or cracks easily. Features with moving parts and single connection points, such as sand diggers, some rockers, and items with handles or mallets, break down often and eventually are not replaced. Wood as a material choice for play equipment, other structures, or landscape features can be more inexpensive to install but presents a big challenge and high cost for long-term maintenance. Where appropriate, durable paving, such as concrete and pavers, should be considered in lieu of asphalt, packed dirt, or decomposed granite because they better withstand high volumes of foot and vehicular traffic in all weather conditions and are far easier for anyone using a mobility device to navigate. With this being said, if resources are available to replace items and materials that provide crucial value to the play space, their most robust versions should be identified and always considered for use.

Build strategies to address vandalism and inappropriate use of amenities in public settings. Unfortunately, to the detriment of their community and themselves, some people will vandalize, break, and destroy the conveniences given to them in public parks. They will creatively find innumerable ways to accomplish destruction. We have seen slides melted with fire, jackets stuffed into toilet plumbing, concrete picnic tables cracked in half and flipped over, trees pulled out of the ground, and metal poles bent at angles—to name just a few. Discouraging as this is, some measures can be taken to combat (although not eliminate) the impact of destructive behaviors.

Much commercially available equipment is fairly susceptible to vandalism. Try to use robust items: choose equipment that is not made of wood and that has few moving parts; high-grade cables and connections; and is mounted to the surface rather than embedded in footings, so they can be simply replaced if needed. Dance chime products are a good example of how strong, difficult-to-vandalize musical equipment meets multiple sensory needs (auditory, visual, tactile, balance, and body awareness). We address sensory-focused play design guidelines later in this chapter.

As mentioned in the previous paragraph, use durable, robust materials wherever possible. Although not impossible to penetrate, a thick steel cabinet for electrical, irrigation, or computer systems is far more difficult to break into than a thin-gauge aluminum, wood, or plastic cabinet. Install security cameras and bright lighting in and around the play space to help discourage untoward behavior. A broad spectrum of security equipment is available, from fake to highly sophisticated. Security companies and equipment can now monitor in real-time, allowing a security agent to be alerted when someone enters a play space. They can talk to, warn, and converse with the trespasser or vandal. This monitoring has been reported to be far more effective and impactful than simply the presence of security equipment lacking live-time monitoring features.

Consider how exposure to weather and other natural elements will be addressed. Few forces are as relentless or rough as the sun and other weather conditions. When exposed to these forces, bright, vibrant, and beautiful quickly become dull, weathered, and ordinary. For the most part, this is inevitable. However, with proper planning, the process can be slowed.

- When selecting finishes and coatings, pick those with longevity. Examples include UV-stable powder coatings, plastics, and rubber surfaces. Avoid purples and yellows because they tend to fade more quickly than other colors.
- When possible, cover key features or equipment under a shade structure, shade sail, or other shading devices. These will also protect against ultraviolet degradation and rain and water damage.
- Equipment for utilities and infrastructure could be placed in restroom chases or other structures instead of outdoors.
- When selecting finishes and colors for pavement or metal structures, consider natural patinas, such as Corten Steel and the Natina coloring system; integral (not topical) coloring systems like Butterfield and Solomon colors; and natural stone because their colors last longer and are more stable.

Building public facilities costs much more than privately funded projects. It is important to consider the landowner and financial mechanisms by which the project will be built. Private fundraising can be a long and difficult process but affords more flexibility during construction. Many US states and jurisdictions require a minimum pay rate for construction and trade laborers working on publicly funded projects or land owned by a public agency. This pay rate, referred to as the "prevailing wage," is typically much higher than the broader legislated minimum wage. Thus, construction costs will increase when a municipality is involved with funding a project due to the requirement to pay prevailing wages.

In addition, if municipal or agency land or resources are involved, the project typically undergoes a public design-bid-build process. This process requires a lengthier course of public requests for design proposals; council and board approvals; often environmental documentation; multidepartment plan reviews, revisions, and resubmittals; and a public bid process to select a contractor. All this takes time and money and can significantly increase the project timeline. Completing a project with private funds is certainly faster and less expensive.

However, using public mechanisms has advantages, as well. Many grants to fund projects are available only to public agencies; these can be substantial and, sometimes, the only way to realize a project. A local jurisdiction may also have land or a site within an existing park available. Not needing to purchase land saves valuable monetary resources for the play space itself. In addition—and depending on the local agency and jurisdiction—staff may have previously completed similar projects and possess expertise that can be very helpful in navigating the process of securing grant funds, producing a design, and ultimately constructing the play space.

Maintenance crews are typically hampered by their schedules, availability, and departmental budget limitations. Thus, they cannot frequently maintain public parks. It takes a great deal of effort to (at a minimum) keep a park and its amenities clean and free of litter, particularly after weekends and holidays when families and friends swarm the parks for picnics, barbeques, and birthday parties. Furthermore, every park requires additional maintenance depending on the amenities provided. As maintenance-intense features, restrooms, high-use sports fields, engineered wood-fiber play surfacing, sand play, and water play can add tremendous time demands to the maintenance schedule. Even though some features, like play structures and rubber surfacing, appear to be low maintenance, they require regular maintenance to remain functional. For example, rubber surfacing needs surface treatment every couple of years, and high-use areas need frequent replacement because the wear layers will thin and unravel.

With generous or sufficient funding endowments from sources like homeowner associations, community facilities districts, or landscape maintenance districts, parks and play spaces can include some higher maintenance intense features. These features should come with the understanding that there will be associated support labor and replacement parts to keep them in good functioning condition. Often, money is not allocated to maintain equipment. Thus, when equipment is vandalized or wears down, it is not replaced. This results in scenarios where swing sets have no seats or chains, play structures have no slides but just boarded-up decks, clear plastic panels are foggy and translucent, and only remnants of the foundations of rockers and spinners are visible. However, many parks throughout the United States are funded through general fund accounts, meaning they do not have dedicated funds associated with their upkeep. Thus, myriad community needs compete with park maintenance needs for limited resources. As a result, park maintenance needs are too commonly deferred first because other community needs are perceived as more critical.

Health Care Facilities

Health care facilities have specific and often rigorous safety and infection control requirements requiring careful attention when planning an inclusive play space. Vector control for mammals, birds, insects, or other arthropods that transmit disease pathogens is of particular concern so that patients are not exposed to other diseases they could contract by being outdoors. An example of vector control is when water play is introduced into the play space. There should be no standing water in the surrounding environment to manage mosquitoes, which can transmit diseases such as the West Nile virus or Dengue fever. However, during water play, manipulative and dynamic play experiences are enriched by damming, stopping, and pooling the water. One possible method of bridging the conflict between no standing water and purposefully collecting water in tubs, bins, and low spots is to incorporate stoppers, flaps, and damming devices that are not entirely waterproof. Instead, they leak enough water to allow for consolidated water during active use and drain out completely when not in use.

Another common form of vector control is incorporating plant species that deter vectors by generating natural deterrents, repellents, toxins, and regulators as defense and protection mechanisms. Examples include highly fragrant plants, such as basils, thymes, catnip, and lemon eucalyptus. Notably, however, not all vectors react equally to plant defense mechanisms. Thus, the selection of plant species should be targeted at the vectors of most concern. For example, catnip has been used in homeopathic remedies as a mosquito repellent; however, it could have the opposite effect by attracting feral cats. As the plant species are being chosen, it is also important to recognize how people are affected by highly aromatic plants. Fragrant plants may severely affect those with sensory processing disorders or undergoing chemotherapy. Thus, great care should be taken to select appropriate plants and locate them in the best areas.

Environmental allergies can be exacerbated for patients with lowered and compromised immune systems. Thoughtful design about the types of plants to use in the play space is important. A great resource to understand what types of plants are most problematic and which are not is the Ogren Plant Allergy Scale. This allergy scale for plants is found in the book *Allergy-Free Gardening: The Revolutionary Guide to Healthy Landscaping* by Thomas Leo Ogren. Although not a completely comprehensive index of all plants, the content provides an allergy rating for many species found in common landscapes. It also offers instructions on how to determine on your own what a plant's general allergy scale might be. In general, male or monoecious plants that are wind pollinated (and thus have light powdery pollen) are detrimental for people with environmental allergies (grasses, oaks, conifers, etc.). Contrarily, flowery and showy plants tend to have heavier sticky pollen that will readily attach to pollinator species like bees. Thus, their pollen does not remain in the air as long, so these plants (hibiscus, sage, periwinkle, etc.) are generally less detrimental to people with allergies.

Emergencies can happen anywhere, including outside in the play space. Installing emergency communication infrastructure is frequently required. In our experience, most hospital management teams prefer installing outdoor phones with hardwire connections at frequent intervals along campus paths and trails to ensure safety and rapid response times. Call boxes and other infrastructure should be highly visible, unobscured, and frequently checked to ensure they are in working order.

Access to the play space in a health care facility differs from other types of facilities. Patients, their families, and other visitors may have various health conditions, be they temporary or ongoing, that require the use of mobility devices or medical equipment such as IV poles. Clear, level, and (vertically and horizontally) unobstructed walkways accommodate this type of equipment and enable patients and their family members to use the play space most easily. Paths with less than ¼-inch grout space between paving materials are essential so IV poles, walkers, and cane tips, and even high heels do not get caught and lead to trip-and-fall situations. Think about a child or adult entering an above-ground play structure or cozy space installed under the structure. Is there enough vertical clearance for an IV pole? Is there enough room to get by another person who might be pulling that IV pole or just learning how to navigate in a wheelchair or using a walker or crutches?

Low-effort walkway grades can make more comfortable and equitable experiences. This crucial consideration will also go a long way toward reducing stress and anxiety. Patients and their families will appreciate getting to and from the play space and being there without adding to the uncertainty and fear of being in a health care facility environment. The US designation for a travel-way ramp is a 5.00%–8.33% slope. However, that much slope is certainly not comfortable and would not be considered low effort. If providing travel paths to higher elevations, stick to paths with less than 5% slopes when feasible. These are not only more comfortable for the user but also easier and safer to traverse—and there is no requirement to provide handrails or guards.

Further, for easily navigated walkways, include several inviting areas to stop along the way, designed to offer a range of calming places—for peace, quiet, or reflection. This is vital in a health care facility type of outdoor environment. These types of spaces might be manifested as small nooks furnished with a table and chairs and easy access for wheelchair companion seating. Families can gather and be together. There may also be small, well-defined spaces that enable people to be alone to read, draw, or meditate.

Controlled access may also be a priority for some institutions. With modern safety and privacy concerns, health care facilities often limit access to their facilities. They sometimes require entry through a secure building or gated entrances. When free and open access is not allowed, it is important to consider how people will come in and out of spaces. In some jurisdictions, an outdoor gate is regarded as a door. As such, it must meet door codes and be equipped with levers, panic bars, kick plates, and clearance zones. Controlled access can also provide a level of protection to outdoor play spaces from which public play spaces do not benefit. It more easily allows incorporating loose parts into the outdoor play environment and even having volunteer or staff docents direct play events. Lastly, families that require very close oversight may be able to enjoy a controlled play space where health care staff can monitor them easily. Without that ability, families might not be allowed to venture outdoors together.

Educational Settings

Educational facility play spaces are often quasi-public spaces. They are closed to the public during school hours and may be open after school until early evening and on weekends. Considerations such as rigorous, high use of amenities by students and other visitors translates into the need for planning and budgeting for ongoing equipment maintenance and replacement. Schoolyard play spaces are some of the most heavily used play areas. When school is in session, the equipment is used all day, every day. Where the play space is open to the public, the local community uses the equipment in the evenings and on weekends. The wear and tear from this frequent and high-intensity use is significant; thus, facilities and management staff desire only the most durable equipment. Items with moving parts, such as gliding tracks, spinners, rockers, and sand diggers, are the most susceptible to this high level of use; hence, they are the first items to break and fall into disrepair. When the play value afforded by these equipment types is desired, make sure a budget is in place for frequent replacement.

Consider installing fencing and locks, which help reduce or deter vandalism and inappropriate use of amenities, and address user safety. Next to the frequency of use, vandalism in play spaces is another significant issue. Vandalism tends to occur most frequently during hours without on-site supervision, so measures intended to discourage unsupervised access to the play space can be effective. Limiting access by installing fencing with locked gates around the school can be one solution to this challenge. However, views differ on the appropriateness of closing facilities to the public that paid taxes to build them. This is a complex issue not addressed in this book. Using security (or faux security) cameras, maintaining visual corridors by locating the play space in a location visible from the road by police, and lighting the area with motion-sensor-equipped dimmer lights can be effective strategies for deterring mischievous behavior after hours.

Budgets are almost always a concern. School districts work perpetually with community groups and parent–teacher organizations to fundraise for a multitude of educational programs, field trips, and curricula they want to provide to the children. Rarely are those efforts geared toward improving the school's outdoor play spaces. With this reality in mind, finding ways to minimize project costs while maximizing play value when working within schoolyards on inclusive play spaces is often important. Some of the many examples of how this might be accomplished include:

- Minimizing earthwork (digging down or building up) by grading the site as close to existing elevations as possible because this is costly work
- Capitalizing on existing shade structures or shade trees by placing play equipment near them
- Utilizing cooperative purchasing programs, like Sourcewell, GSA, or HGACBuy, to avoid contractor markups and get the best deals on equipment
- Minimizing flatwork and hardscape because it can be one of the most expensive components of site work

- Considering locating play spaces near utility connections, such as storm drains and water, minimizing long utility extensions and connection costs
- Considering an aggregate rather than a concrete base when using unitary surfacing

School maintenance crews often do not have the time or expertise to maintain play spaces to the highest level needed for ongoing use and intense use (or "abuse"). Standards are in place in the United States to determine whether play spaces are safe. The NRPA has developed a certification to regulate who can review play spaces for safety conformance. These individuals are referred to as *certified playground safety inspectors* (CPSIs). Due to the cost and time associated with becoming a CPSI, schools typically do not have anyone on staff to determine whether their play spaces meet minimum standards. As a result, many play spaces remain in unsafe condition because safety surfacing is not thick enough or does not provide enough cushioning; S-hooks for swings are worn down and in danger of breaking; gaps have formed between slides and the rest of the play structure, causing a potential snag location; or many other issues exist.

School district risk managers may not allow some of the play features found in public parks, such as swings or spinners, to be included in school play spaces. Many times over the years, I (Chad) have met with risk managers who quoted from the CPSI training class literature on the types of play equipment with the highest associated rates of injury and death. As a result of their interpretation of this data, they frequently ban their use in district facilities.

Be aware that the concern about installing these play features despite the risk being mitigated with proper design and planning exists. Banning these features ignores the children's developmental needs to swing and spin.

Joint use agreements with municipalities or other organizations can result in complications. As is often the case, school districts and municipalities operate independently of one another and are regulated separately. However, the open spaces each create can be valuable assets to the other party. For example, if a city builds a baseball complex near a high school, the school may elect not to build its own fields. Instead, they use the city fields as their practice and game fields. Conversely, if a school builds open grass fields in an area lacking open space, the city may use the school's fields for youth sports outside operating hours. In both cases, the parties benefit from each other by utilizing the same space. This is often done with facilities such as pools, sports fields, auditoriums, and even inclusive play spaces. In California, one such project received funding from a school district. They agreed that the district had exclusive rights to use the public park at certain times of the day and week for their special education class field trips. Complications with these agreements can arise, however, as the agreements are negotiated—and not always successfully. Some of the many complications might include the following:

- Politics sometimes get in the way. Significant hurdles and obstacles to finding workable solutions could arise without a good working relationship between the municipality and school district stakeholders.
- Determining a schedule for when each group can use the facility might become a challenge. Schools have outdoor activities, festivals, and events outside typical school hours that might overlap municipal sports leagues and other uses.
- Determining who maintains and pays for maintenance of the open space can become a significant sticking point. Either party might dispute the potential monetary value of their impact on the space.
- In many cases, a rental or lease agreement is put in place for the use of the space. Landing a fair deal for both sides is often a challenge.
- The length of the rental or lease term may not work for either party. One might want a long-term commitment, and the other may want or need a shorter one.
- One party may require certain upgrades to the facility at the other's cost to meet the needs of their intended use. Examples include adding parking, fencing around restrooms, or ADA upgrades.

Guidelines for Play Strategies

Most people who visit a play space have no idea of the thought and care that has gone into its design. A well-crafted inclusive[+] design is developed by an interdisciplinary design team that takes into account all the design principles noted in Chapter 6, "Inclusive Design." The team finds creative ways to marry the principles with any play area and user group's opportunities and constraints. There is no limit to the innovative approaches that can be explored or generated in response to future research and evaluation of inclusive play spaces. As researchers and designers actively engaged in the design process, we have seen many amazing ideas, concepts, and strategies develop over the years. We eagerly look forward to what more is to come. The following are just a few of the innovative and impactful strategies and implementation techniques we use and have seen used in inclusive[+] play space design.

Independent Play

Independent play is an experience where children have chances to learn skills that will support independence, such as decision-making, confidence, self-reliance, and resilience (Murniyati & Wardhani, 2023; Sunarty & Dirawan Darma, 2015). Design can support independent play by providing the features discussed in this section.

Accessible/Traversable Surfaces

If a play area is difficult to travel through, it limits a child's ability to determine on their own where they will go and what they will do. There are many ways to plan for all-weather accessible and traversable surfaces that will support independent movement around the play space. Using solid, stable materials, like concrete, pavers, asphalt, and, when correctly installed, stabilized decomposed granite, will provide long-term, reliable access to, and movement through and between play areas.

When planning for surfaces within the play areas, impact attenuation and stability for accessibility must be jointly considered. The most common stable and accessible attenuation materials are PIP rubber surfacing and rubber tiles/mats. However, other materials can be used successfully and similarly, but have their pros and cons. Some of these materials include a new cork-based PIP product installed like PIP rubber surfacing, but it is a natural, renewable product. Play carpet, specifically developed for outdoor play scenarios, is underlaid with an attenuation layer. Another option is artificial turf, which is available in many colors, pile heights, and configurations. Notably, it is also underlaid with an attenuation layer. Combitile® is similar to rubber tiles but with a unique, separate underlay system, making it ideal for wet and dry applications. When installed with natural grass, rubber grass mats offer a unique way to maintain natural grass in a play space while providing a stable and attenuating surface.

Confined Play Areas

Confinement of play areas creates reliable and safe boundaries within the play space so independent play can transpire. These physical boundaries provide caregivers with increased security to allow their children to roam and explore on their own terms. In particular, children prone to wandering, bolting, or running away (also referred to as elopement) during incidents of sensory overload benefit from the security of confined play areas. In confined or enclosed play areas, children at risk for elopement can run freely to refuge without their caregivers giving chase. This safety feature allows children to determine where they need to go and what they need to do to return to a state of regulation and calmness. These barriers are not intended to keep people out of the area; rather, they keep people in. The most common way of achieving this goal is with trap fences that are only 4 feet tall. Although 6 feet is a standard fence height, a 4-foot fence is sufficient to slow a child attempting to leave the play space.

Fences are often used because they are commonly available, visually permeable, difficult to vandalize, easy to maintain, and have proven longevity. For similar reasons, solid walls are widely used. They effectively block sound but are expensive to construct, easily vandalized, and not visually permeable. Other less common options might include vegetated hedges, which are maintenance heavy and may not have complete coverage but are more attractive than structural solutions. Cable and post systems are visually unobtrusive and provide a less solid barrier than other methods. Glass/plastic/metal panels can be customized and add play and sensory value to the play space's theme, but they are costly. Steep mounds or hills, which slow a child's intention to leave the space, can also be considered.

Accessible Equipment

Perhaps one of the most important ways to encourage self-empowerment is by providing complete access to all parts of the play area, separate and independent from caregivers. We believe that to be considered inclusive[+], all areas, in particular the highest location of the play space, should be completely accessible for every child, regardless of any type of assistive or ambulatory device. Access to higher elevations is achievable in most conditions by using ramps with grades between 5.00% and 8.23%. However, to limit unintended and unnecessary physical exertion and align with the universal design principle of low physical effort, it is ideal to design ramps, walkways, and access ways with grades less than 5.00%. This ensures that everyone has the opportunity to reach high spaces.

When ramps must be installed, they can be enhanced with playful, sensory-rich, and interactive features, like roller ball and abacus panels. This consideration helps make the journey to the apex of the play space a more interesting, stigma-free experience and less of a challenge to overcome. Play equipment, panels, signs, and interactive play elements should be set at reach-range heights from sitting to standing positions for maximum flexibility and usability.

Another key inclusive[+] feature is limiting the required effort to activate or use the interactive play equipment. This is accomplished by providing handles, knobs, or activating devices that do not require refined fine-motor skills but can be used with a larger whole-hand grasp. Other strategies include using large, extruded buttons to push with the entire palm or elbow and selecting products with ball bearings that move smoothly and without friction. These are great ways to ensure that children can play independently without assistance from a caregiver (see Figure 7.1).

Another way to support independence through accessibility is to use multisensory forms of communication on signs or elsewhere in the play space. This includes Brailling signs and using raised and embossed lettering so those who are visually challenged can read on their own. Another option is to provide tactile cues along the path of travel, clearly indicating how to get to each section of the play area and its amenities. For younger children who cannot read, and to promote equity for all, easily understood simple icons and recognizable symbols are representative of inclusive[+] design.

Cause and Effect

Children learn the consequences of actions they take through play with elements fundamentally geared around interactive play. Learning consequences in a safe and forgiving environment is integral to childhood development. Cause-and-effect

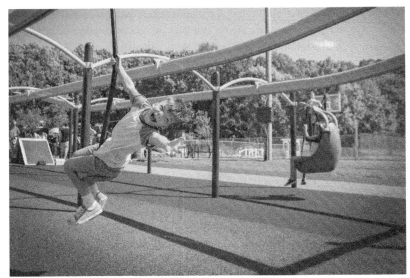

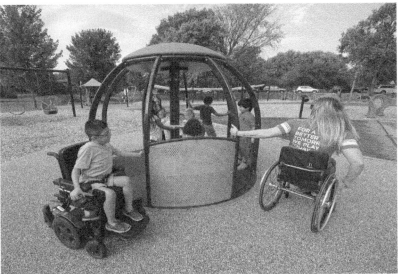

FIGURE 7.1 Examples of manufactured inclusive play elements that provide vestibular input, motion, and fun. Credit- Landscape Structures Inc.

experiences can be introduced into a play space in many creative ways. The following are a few ideas to get you thinking:

- Mechanical game panels, like marble mazes, gear cog panels, and color-changing wheels, afford children opportunities to move pieces or knobs and immediately see the resulting change from their actions. These types of play elements are well suited for repetition and revision to achieve different results, playing over and over again.

- Similarly, in a controlled and monitored environment, vertically oriented manipulation walls filled with door handles of different sizes and shapes, wheels, hinges, buttons, switches, and the like provide real-world applications for decision-making. For example, what happens when you open a door? When you flip a switch, what happens next?

- A modern twist to mechanical panels is electronic play panels. They often require a child to generate the energy necessary to power the panel. The effort sustained may reinforce the consequence of the actions taken. A series of vibrations, sounds, or lights can result from selecting options like tripping sensors and pushing buttons. Some are available as adaptive switch capable, thus increasing inclusiveness.

- Musical instruments, such as chimes and drums, can also be an effective way to experience cause and effect: When an instrument is struck or hit with hands or a mallet, pleasant or unpleasant sounds/music can be produced.

- Loose-parts play items are one of the best ways to provide children with opportunities to control their immediate environment. However, as effective and fun as loose parts play may be, it can be a challenge in public play settings. Unfortunately, typical loose-play items, such as buckets, tools, balls, and fabricated play systems, like Snug Play or Imagination Playground®, tend to disappear or be stolen. We found that natural elements are the most effective way to provide loose play in public spaces. It is important to consider that sand and water play features—although sometimes requiring high maintenance—are excellent and beloved childhood materials for loose play, particularly when combined. In the spirit of inclusive[+] design, when including sand and water play in a play space, be sure to provide them at elevated levels (not just at ground level) so everyone can enjoy it. (Other nature-based items ideal for loose-parts play are described in the upcoming Nature-Based Play section) (see Figure 7.2).

Cognitive Simplicity

Simple, easy-to-understand spaces help reduce confusion and provide a comfortable space conducive to independent exploration. If a child feels lost or unsure of where they are, where to go, or what to do, they will unlikely be independent and take the initiative to explore the play space. When a play space is planned to help children and their families create cognitive mental maps, the spaces are more successful. These maps can be "drawn" more readily when there are clear lines of sight into, through, and out of the play area. This means that visual obstructions are minimal but not nonexistent. A simple way to orient oneself is by using readily visible and recognizable landmarks in the play space. These landmarks may be themed, like giant giraffes in a safari-focused play space, clocktowers in a city-focused play space, or windmills and flowers that are highly visible from most areas of the play space.

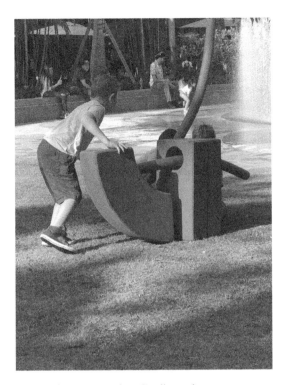

FIGURE 7.2   Cooperative loose parts play. Credit- author.

They also can be less thematic, like unique restroom facilities, consistent way-finding signs, specimen trees, or tall play structures. Ample sweeping curves in the travel ways in lieu of windy, tight paths are more understandable. When designed in tandem with a pathway hierarchy of widths and surfaces, these curves can simplify navigation of the space. Path hierarchies may be developed so that major pathways are wide but start to narrow where offshoot paths access smaller areas. Surface materials, colors, and textures, such as broom-finish concrete, stamped concrete, asphalt, stone or concrete pavers, and attenuating surfaces, may be changed to emphasize transitions into new spaces further or alert visitors that they are leaving the play space.

Design teams can create distinctly recognizable areas within a play space by theming through equipment content, plant palette selection, and color coordination. An example of this is the Awesome Spot Playground in Modesto, California (see case study at Chapter 4, Box 4.3), where the three play space areas were themed separately: Savanna Safari (for 2- to 5-year-olds), Rain Forest Excursion (5- to 12-year-olds), and Swamp Cruise (transition high-activity area). The play equipment in each area has a bend toward its theme, such as animal climbers, distinctive steel baobab tree-art landmarks, large tropical leaf shade covers, and boat rockers. The plants within each area were also chosen to match the theme. Plants in the savanna are geared more toward arid plant communities; those in the rain forest showcase larger leaves and flowers; and the swamp incorporates interesting rushes and reeds. Even the attenuating surfaces are designed to emphasize the themes. The savanna area is heavy in tans and browns, the rain forest with deep greens and rich browns, and the swamp with shades of blue. Visitors can readily orient themselves regardless of where they are in this large play space.

Dramatic Play

Younger children particularly need safe environments to reenact the events that play out around them. The reenacting process, often called *dramatic play*, is one way children learn to make decisions on their own and interact with people and the built environment. Opportunities for dramatic play do not need to be prescriptive in design decisions: When given a chance, children can use their creativity to change the world around them. Light and simple suggestions, such as playhouses, shop-window panels, faux cash registers, outdoor kitchens, automobile gas pumps, artistic murals, raised platforms or stages, and themed play elements, can prompt dramatic play. The May Nissen Playground in Livermore, California, is an example of a creative approach to dramatic play (see case study, Box 7.1). A small story nook (fairy-tale-themed play space) was installed off to the side of the play area.

The play space has a 12-inch high stage accessed by a low-effort walkway to the side. The stage can be used for impromptu reenactments or musical shows for people of all ages. It has several rows of benches for spectators and multiple features that support storytelling and music. When wound up, an interactive story ball in one corner plays recorded audible stories. Next to the stage, a child-powered speaker amplifies anyone's smartphone speaker so that everyone can hear the teller's story or music. To add to all these wonderful features, several types of tuned percussion instruments on the stage encourage anyone, with or without musical skills, to recreate the music they love for all to hear.

Centennial Park in Madera, California (see case study, Box 7.2), has a perimeter path that emulates a drive through California's poppy fields, complete with rolling mounds, larger-than-life poppy flowers, a gas station, a motorcycle rocker ride-on toy, and other California-focused stops along the way. With such a varied range of options, children can make their own decisions about how they will play and what they will reenact through their dramatic play.

Creativity and Exploration

When a child feels safe and secure in a space, they are more likely to venture further from caregivers. They sometimes even like being "hidden" from them. This simultaneous feeling of safety, security, and autonomy can inspire a sense of exploration and curiosity within them. When well planned, a play space can and should encourage exploration. If on the hierarchy of paths, small offshoot paths lead to more intimate spaces—with maybe small shrubs or other obstacles that obstruct a child's view but not necessarily the caregiver's—these spaces can catalyze creative, exploratory behaviors. It is even more relevant when coupled with natural elements and games that require searching.

At Sunridge Park in Rancho Cordova, California, a network of accessible but narrower paths along the play space perimeter and within wide areas of no-mow grass designed with an earthy color tone leads to seven different gathering areas. Within each gathering spot is a hidden marking of a native animal species. On the play structure nearby is a seek-and-find panel and a telescope through which each animal marking can be identified from afar and then discovered from below, along the path. There are also many types of plants and flowers along the path to observe and explore. Another way to encourage children to be independent through creative exploration is to embed different kinds of visually interesting, tactile items into the bottom or walls of sand beds/pits to be excavated and discovered by children as they dig.

Looping

If you have ever had the pleasure of swinging an infant around like an airplane, over and over and over again, because they just cannot get enough of it, you can relate to the value children place on repeating an activity. The play space is no exception to promoting opportunities for repetitive play. Thus, play space design must be purposeful in its placement of activities to allow and encourage looping cycles. The most common way to accomplish looping on a play structure is to locate the exit of a slide chute near a transition station or entry point back into the structure. Circular paths leading back to the original start point—with activities or offshoots of grouped play elements along the way—are also unique, fun ways to loop activities and enhance the creativity factor.

Intuitive Spaces and Clear Delineations

When play spaces are intuitive, children do not need to expend energy or worry about navigation. They can just play. This is important! Children should be afforded opportunities for independent play rather than spend their time assessing dangerous situations and trying to avoid getting lost. During a recent visit to a play space touted as inclusive in the greater metro Seattle, Washington area, we observed that a train track had been integrated into the rubber surfacing throughout the play area. This was a fun idea, but we found an issue with its implementation. The train track, which children follow instinctively as a pathway (Chad knows firsthand because he did it without thinking), leads right into active use zones—of the swings in one location and an elevated spinner in another—before finally terminating in the grass lawn. This is a dangerous and confusing example of how *not* to make a space intuitive or clear. It is anything but.

Conversely, an inclusive[+] play space project can be designed using colors and strategic placement to indicate where activity is occurring and how it can be avoided. Red, universally viewed as the color for stop or danger, can identify slides, swings, spinners, and other active features. These features also should be oriented away from paths of travel to avoid unintended conflicts. The color blue is often associated with water. Using it to denote drinking fountains, splash pads, water play, and other water representations is another way to identify the elements within a play space clearly. Selecting and embedding a clear hierarchy of colors and shapes in the rubber surfacing under and around the active features can effectively deter runners through the space and avoid accidents. For instance, a play space recently installed at Valley Children's Hospital in Madera, California is based on an agricultural theme. It included a clump of grapes on a vine to delineate the safety zone of the swings and a sack of corn at a slide chute to delineate the exit region. Children quickly accommodate to cues like this (see Figure 7.3).

Social Play

Engaging in cooperative activities and group games in a play space are effective methods to encourage positive social interaction between children and, as appropriate, the adults in their lives (Wenger et al., 2021). Social play can be encouraged through the features discussed in the following paragraphs.

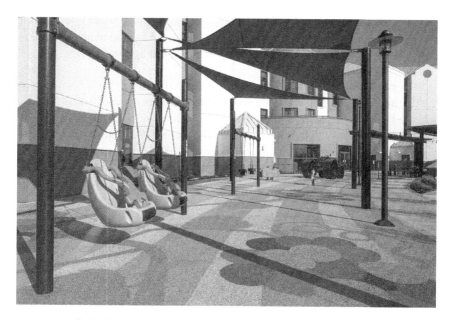

FIGURE 7.3   Surfacing can serve as a visual safety cue. Credit- author.

Cozy Spaces

Children may need time to acclimate to the play space or take a break. Cozy spaces near the action and on the periphery of the play space provide much-needed opportunities for self-regulation and self-determination regarding when they are ready to jump back into active play. These cozy spaces can also be a great transition zone between play spaces of differing types, like active, highly sensory-based, or passive activities. A cozy space can be created with manufactured equipment, like the Cozy Dome®, Cozy Cocoon®, or crawl tubes, but do not necessarily need to be manufactured items. Spaces under decks or ramps or small spaces designed into the landscape can be just as effective. Cozy spaces should be designed in conjunction with prospect and refuge theory principles to be small, tighter spaces where more than one side of the body can contact a surface and provide good visibility of the surroundings with some texture on surfaces to create tactile interest.

Cooperative Play (Multiuser Equipment)

Playing with other children should be a naturally occurring process, not forced upon them. The environment can hinder playing together when only single-user-type activities are provided. Thus, planning opportunities that encourage children to interact with peers in all types of play is vital. Incorporating multiuser capacity features can suggest to families that playing together as a family or with other children is okay. Items like disc swings are large enough to accommodate multiple users and more fun with additional people. Swings of this type can be found in many public play spaces. Water taps and pumps that are hard to maintain the flow and capture water at the same time also encourage collaborative play.

> *At a park grand opening a few years ago, Chad's son was playing on a motorcycle spring rocker specifically chosen because it has a small sidecar with attached postural support for multiuser play. As he played on it, a young toddler, he did not know walked by, observed what he was doing, and, without a word, climbed up into the sidecar. They had a great time together, and their play continued to other areas of the play space. This is an excellent example of how the play environment and play elements can suggest but not prescribe play.*

Electronic play equipment has opened up other avenues for cooperative play. Electronic play can be structured around collaborative challenges as a team or in competition with another person, even from different areas of the play space.

Auditory Expression and Listening

Social interactions rely on communication, be it verbal, sign language, picture boards, or electronic systems. Here we explore strategies to encourage and incorporate auditory communication. Play spaces should incorporate opportunities to use real or simulated (via electronic communication devices) voices during play. This might include installing talk tubes in multiple locations throughout the play space.

The Addy Grace playground in Daleville, Virginia (see case study at Chapter 6, Box 6.1), has a maze of talk tubes that create a fun game of trying to locate the tubes that connect to each other. For some children and adults, experiencing echoes can be a fun way to explore verbal expression. Echo chambers can be created for this, such as one installed at the Boulder, Colorado Sensory Garden. Updated versions of the talk tube now integrate multiple pipes, creating a compounded echo effect that alters vocalizations, encouraging exploration of the different ways to use one's voice. An interesting natural play piece from Europe, the Singing Stone, uses cavities carved in stone to encourage exploring one's voice. The Lerner Garden of the Five Senses at the Coastal Maine Botanical Garden has multiheight naturalized stone talking tubes that children and adults widely enjoy. These singing stones and talking tubes encourage music-making, singing, humming, and adjusting one's pitch so it reverberates within the natural stone.

A more passive approach to verbal exchange and conversation is parabolic reflectors. These devices can be integrated into seats or placed in different locations (even up to 100 feet or more away) to encourage exploration of sound with others, from a distance. Some play space users feel comfortable vocalizing within the larger play space; others will feel comfortable using their voice when it is just them and another individual or in a small group. Inclusive[+] design acknowledges this range of comfort. It creates small areas for gathering in an offshoot of the path or a circular fashion. A cluster of rocks, one or two benches, or a couple of strategically placed tree stumps can be just enough to do the trick and encourage less gregarious people to converse on their terms.

Eye-Level Play

As a matter of the human condition, communicating at eye level with others removes an unconscious perception of superiority, intimidation, inequality, and lack of acceptance. It replaces these negative perceptions with feelings of safety, control, and connection. Communicating at eye level helps convey that you are interested in communicating *with*—not at or about—them. This is particularly important for wheeled mobility users who far too often are spoken to from above. Why should a child or adult who uses a wheeled mobility device have to literally look up to their standing counterpoint when being spoken to? Conversely, how inequitable is it for the person standing to look down upon someone seated?

Creating play options where children can play at eye level with each other can mitigate some of this inequity in the play environment. Raised sand, water, or planters with roll-under capacity that are ADA compliant are great for this. One child can play with the raised play element while standing, while a child who is seated plays from the side at the same eye level. Companion seat benches and tables or spaces between benches where a wheelchair or stroller can roll in are also effective ways to seat people next to each other equitably. Where there is an activity panel or feature, make certain there is roll-under capacity so that seated and standing children can play together in an inclusive⁺ manner.

Parallel Play

A component of social play is the option to play alongside another person doing the same thing, regardless of whether an interaction occurs. Although an ultimate goal is connections and shared play experiences between children, parallel play is a starting point (refer to Chapter 3, "History and Value of Outdoor Play," for a more detailed discussion of parallel play). Inclusive⁺ play spaces attempt to create situations where, when needed, all play can be both parallel and interactive. It can be achieved by selecting double-wide roller slides or duo/triple track slides so more than one child can experience sliding motion at the same time. When planning for swings, alternate between belt seats and chair seats so there is no difference or separation between a user's needs. If musical equipment is desired, include multiple similar features near each other to be used in tandem. Make ramps to access greater heights double-wide so children can traverse them together. Games can even be incorporated along the rampways for added parallel play opportunities.

Social Pods

Not long ago, I (Chad) assisted a small elementary charter school with the design of a play space for their campus. During an on-site design team visit, I was shocked when an administrator divulged that they do not allow children to sit in groups, read, or engage in other passive recreation during recess. Their policy was to force children to play actively, hence burning energy and, in theory, improving in class behavior.

Unfortunately, this policy did not consider each child's differing social and sensory needs. The right balance of social and active sensory input is not the same for all children. Forced moderate-to-vigorous physical activity (often referred to as MVPA) can be the opposite of what some children need. An appropriate and inclusive⁺ approach to meet the diverse needs for social interaction would be to provide social gathering spaces of varied sizes. Large and smaller, more intimate groups could accommodate active, dramatic, quiet, or social play.

We recently saw two teenagers playing their guitars in a park. They were sitting on top of an electrical equipment box sited away from everyone. This was probably not an ideal place to "hang out," but it was all they had available to them.

*If this park had provided more spaces for small groups, those teenagers could
have had a much more enjoyable experience.*

Research out of Utah State University showed a strong correlation between the
highest elevation of a play space and the amount of social interaction that occurs.
The higher children go, the more they interact. With this in mind—and because
more social interaction occurs at the highest elevations—the most enjoyable and
desirable activities should be located at the highest elevation, as long as access
is easy and equal for *all* children. That is the approach taken at EmPOWERment
Park (see case study, Box 7.2), where play decks at 12-foot elevations were intentionally oversized to accommodate more children and the highest concentration of
activities, like an interactive team-based game, child-powered ceiling fans, musical
chimes, and access to a tube slide.

Affect Attunement

Closely related to eye-level play, affective emotional exchange occurs between
young children and adults when they gaze face-to-face at each other (Jongerius
et al., 2020; Niedźwiecka, 2020). This nonverbal exchange helps form secure attachment relationships (Farroni et al., 2002). It is the beginning of learning the
dance of how to share emotional experiences, a critical element of social interaction. This often intimate, face-to-face experience can be created in the play space
through activities that occur in close proximity.

Recently, many caregiver–toddler swings have been introduced to the market.
These situate a child swing directly in front of an adult seat, so they face each other
as they swing. Important in selecting a swing is it forgiving the movements adults
might make—jerky movements can create an uncomfortable ride for children with
limited upper-body strength and control or vestibular challenges. Of note are some
adult–child swing versions with hard plastic or metal connections between seats.
These have been shown to be a conduit for misuse, causing the entire swing to fail
and requiring repeated replacements.

Another clever adaptation is a picnic table with a toddler seat embedded in the
tabletop. The child can sit up high and close to the caregiver. Elevated view panels
and translucent bubbles that can be accessed from both sides also can support affect
attunement. The caregiver can look into the panel from the low side as the child
plays at the higher level.

Graduating Levels of Complex Play

By design, the play space and its elements contain a hierarchy of motor, cognitive, and social-emotional opportunities for children to master (Lifter et al., 1993).
Graduating levels of complex play can be nurtured through the concepts discussed
in this section.

Equality and Flexibility

Everyone has room to grow and learn, and you should design with increasingly challenging activity types and consideration for activity locations within a play space on a continuum of simple to complex: simple (*may require assistance or support*), moderate (*needs less assistance or support*), and complex (*needs no assistance or support*). An example that conveys this principle is grouping play space spinners. A ground-level spinner is an excellent option for children with balance or motor-control challenges. They can sit or lay on the spinner or receive assistance to try to stand on it while it spins. Because it is installed at ground level, the required effort and motor control to spin is less intense.

The next level up in complexity (moderate) might be a raised spinner bowl. Its bowl is deep enough to provide postural support for someone with limited upper-body strength and stability. Because these bowls are typically installed at an angle, the bowl can spin with some movement but without assistance from a peer or adult. With practice, a child can use centrifugal force to keep the bowl moving indefinitely.

An additional level up in complexity (complex) might be a spinner that requires activation from a standing posture. This kind of spinner spins and pivots in multiple directions from a single point, requiring much higher levels of balance and motor control to remain on the device and upright. These more complex spinners are also more conducive to multiuser play, creating even further levels of complex play potential (see Figure 7.4).

Another example of graduating difficulty levels is climbing-related play. A simple example is a short vertical ladder that leads to a deck. The next level in complexity (moderate) might be an arch climber requiring a child to orient their head forward, resulting in a change in body alignment. This is a more difficult movement pattern to manage than a straight up-and-down climb. The next complexity level (complex) might be a rock-climbing wall, where decisions about navigation routes, sizes, types of hand and footholds, and multiple changes of body position in space orientation create a much more challenging climb.

Sometimes a designer can achieve graduating difficulty levels with one play element. The Bankshot™ game is one example. This game comprises several basketball-like hoops and backboards arranged in any number of patterns. The backboards vary in size, shape, and angle: Some hoops are low and simple to throw a ball into, and others are high and very difficult to toss a ball through. Within this one system, those with less strength, range of motion, or shooting skill can practice on easier hoops and eventually work their way up to the more challenging hoops only a few feet away. With regard to the play space site itself, more complex play elements can be located further from the entrance of a play space or accessed via a curvy (versus straight) pathway. Not only is the play element more complex but so is the journey to get to it.

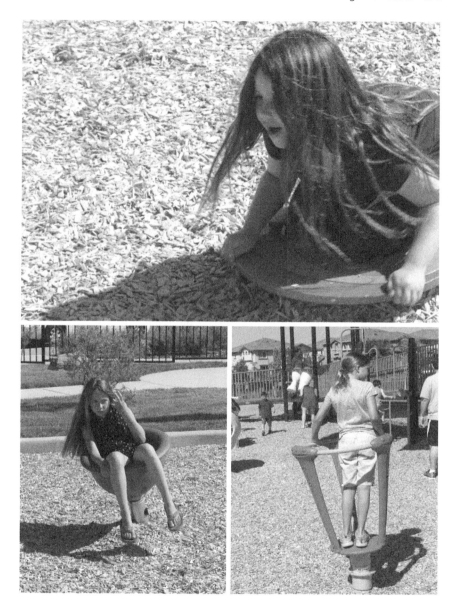

FIGURE 7.4 Example of increasing the challenge in play. Credit- Cordova Recreation and Park District.

Diversity in Play Types

A key principle for inclusive[+] play spaces is acknowledging developmental diversity in play features and activities. To the greatest extent possible, children should be able to find the "just-right" play level they need. This can be challenging, particularly when the construction budget is a primary constraint. Diversity in play opportunities often means additional play areas, surfacing, and equipment. However, it is possible to meet multiple needs with one feature or device.

Recall that children of multiple ages and a wide range of skills, strengths, and mobilities can use a Bankshot™ court. This can be a strategy to minimize costs. One way to determine if a design is diversified enough is to generate an inventory of the design, noting all the purposes for which its features were intended. Once an inventory is in place, evaluating the distribution of play types accounted for in the place space can highlight what deficiencies might exist. At a minimum, an assessment should focus on the many facets of play types, such as physical, cognitive, sensory, and social.

Figure 7.5 illustrates an example of how this might be done, quickly highlighting the relative balance of play needs accounted for and what remains to be addressed. Because any given feature can be intended to achieve multiple play purposes, Figure 7.5 assigns a primary, secondary, and tertiary reason for including each feature. The pie graphs in the upper left-hand corner of the assessment graphically convey to a designer the distribution achieved for overall, primary, and secondary play purposes. When using a tool like this, adjustments can be made early in the planning process, progressing closer to achieving an inclusive⁺ design.

Diversity in Grasping and Gripping

The ability to grasp and hold onto an object and subsequently pull or push it may be challenging for some children and adults. Young children whose fine-motor skills are a work in progress, children and adults with arthritis, children with sensory processing disorder and aversive to certain tactile experiences, and people with limited use of their hands will often find it particularly challenging to use play features that require complex grasping. Thus, it is important to pay particular attention to any access or play feature that requires a handle, rung, or handhold.

Some play panels call for the use of a handle or a hand spinner, like a typical gear panel that moves all the gears when one small gear is twisted with a two-finger pincer motion. These should be modified to be large and easy enough to push with an open hand so that a more complex grasp motion is not required. A fantastic example of this is the Cam Chimes Musical Play Panel. Instead of the typical mallets to play the chimes, this panel uses strikers on each chime that can be easily located and then, with little effort, lifted or patted to strike the chime. A child can grasp the striker for additional impact strength if they want to, but that is unnecessary to engage in playing the chimes. Another example is the Music & Story Ball play equipment, which has a low-energy lever equipped with a large ball at the end. This makes it easy to see and push, so almost everyone can create the kinetic energy needed to hear music or a story.

Project Name: _____ Date: _____

| | Total Primary Purpose Inclusive Activities | Total Secondary Purpose Inclusive Activities: **53** | Total Tertiary Purpose Inclusive Activities: **41** | Total Inclusive Play Opportunities: **20** | **114** |

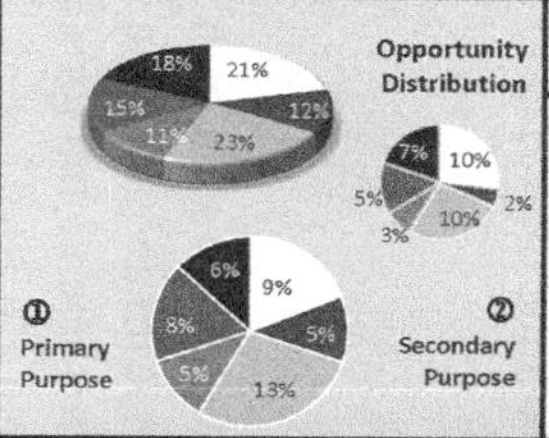

Opportunity Distribution — 77%, 10%, 2%, 10%, 3%, 5%

Primary Purpose — 18%, 21%, 12%, 23%, 15%, 11%

Secondary Purpose — 6%, 9%, 5%, 13%, 5%, 8%

Column categories (left to right):

- **Cognitive Opportunities:** Dramatic, Creativity, Cause & Effect, Exploration, Wayfinding, Looping, Intuitive
- **Basic 5 Sensory Opportunities:** Visual, Auditory, Olfactory, Tactile, Taste, Cozy Spaces
- **Physical Opportunities:** Fine Motor Skills, Gross Motor Skills, Motor Planning, Gravity & Movement, Physical Accessibility, Muscle Tone, Temperature Regulation
- **Interoception Opportunities:** Thirst & Hunger, Non-Sustained Effort (Pain), Tolerance for Error (Pain), Digestive System Impulses, Low Allergens, Awareness
- **Proprioceptive & Vestibular Opportunities:** Balance, Dizziness, Recovery/Rest, Stretching/Compression, Postural Security, Elevation Variation
- **Social Opportunities:** Verbal Expression, Listening, Interaction, Jump-in Point, Independence, User Comfort, Equality/Flexibility in Use

 # PLAYGROUND STRUCTURE EQUIPMENT

#	Item
1	Double Zip Slide
2	Steering Wheel
1	Thespian Theater
2	Wave Climber
1	Curved Slide
4	Crow's Nest w/Telescope
2	Gizmo Panel
3	Schooner Climber
1	Clover Leaf Climber
1	Rockscape
1	Calabazo
1	Music Panel
1	Crunch Bar
1	Rung Enclosure
1	Therapeutic Rings
1	Tree Climber
1	Crazy Eight Climber
1	Climbing Pole
1	Corkscrew Climber
1	Double Seat
1	Wilder Slide
1	Ramps
1	Ramp Curbing
1	Custom Maze Panel

 # STAND ALONE FEATURES

#	Item
1	Tot Swing
2	Bucket seats
1	School-age Swing
1	Ring Swing

FIGURE 7.5 Comprehensive inclusive play environments audit© by Chad Kennedy of O'Dell Engineering. All rights reserved.

Some children will not want to grasp handholds or levers that require them to place the palm of their hand on a surface; this sensory experience can be aversive for them. For this reason, it is preferable to include varied types of play equipment that offer different touch (tactile) experiences. These might slowly enable the children to work up on their terms to a point where they are comfortable making contact with and activating most of the play elements with their whole hand, not just their fingers or fingertips. Instead, they will be ready and less sensorially defensive to using both the fingers and palms of their hands.

Diversity in Physical and Cognitive Effort Levels

Throughout this book, and resonating in this chapter, is the theme that inclusive[+] design means designing for all types of diversity. Here we focus on the physical and mental effort needed to participate in an inclusive[+] play space. All users are seeking a "just-right" level experience that meets their needs. Thus, the design should include some activities and travel ways that are simple and require minimal physical and cognitive effort and others that present a challenge for those who choose to engage with the more difficult options. Whatever the choice, there should never be any shame associated with selecting the less effortful option: Both the simple and the complex options should be designed to be equally fun and engaging.

No matter the simpler or more complex play options, all main pathways that lead to areas of interest and play features should always require low effort (no or limited ramps). However, it is quite appropriate to provide alternate and side routes that offer greater physical and cognitive challenge and exploration of one's abilities, like stepping stone paths, hills with climbing assists, varied height stumps to jump between, spinners like the Supernova, spring rockers, and active court games.

Play features should also require little effort to engage, like water-play tables, large and easily activated electronic buttons on play panels, or smooth paths on a life-size gameboard. Activities with more aggressive effort levels can also be included for those looking for additional challenge. When purposely designing for all options to be easily accessible, give children a choice to determine what they can and want to engage in at that moment and perhaps the next time they visit to challenge themselves to try a more complex activity.

Physical and Risky Play

Physical and risky play help children manage stress, learn to follow through with an activity, improve social interaction skills, increase creativity, learn about human fragility, understand their limitations, recognize areas for improvement, and form positive, proactive attitudes toward others and the environment (Brussoni et al., 2012; Coates & Pimlott-Wilson, 2019; Gleave, 2008; Tai, 2022). We can support physical and risky play through the following activities.

Fine-Motor Activities

Fine-motor skills are enriched through play; likewise, play enhances fine-motor skills. Play features intended to provide opportunities to pinch, grasp, and release and any other activity that uses the hand and fingers can improve children's dexterity and hand–eye coordination. Loose play, in particular, play involving the use of tools, presents a healthy level of risky play when appropriately monitored. Modern electronic game panels and interactive features that involve using the hands and fingers also deliver a level of social risk because they offer opportunities to compete with and against others in the play area. As children engage in what may be outside of their comfort zone, they take risks in learning to negotiate their physical and social boundaries and environment.

Gross-Motor Activities

Activities that promote the use of the larger muscle systems in the trunk, arms, and legs—such as climbing, jumping, pulling, pushing, swinging, hanging, and rolling—in the context of risky play are ways to help children grow stronger and more confident and aware of where their bodies are in space. Gross-motor upper-body activities generally focus on hanging and pushing equipment, like self-powered rotating spinners; monkey bars; a rock wall, horizontal bar, and vertical panel climbers; hand cycles; rope structures; roller tables; and track rides. Gross-motor lower-body activities generally include play features like rocks and boulders, tree stumps, hills, merry-go-rounds, dance chimes, steppers, balance beams, court games, and surface gameboards.

Opportunities for Risk

Children need to push their boundaries in a safe manner to learn and take relative risks based on their comfort level and abilities. However, children should not be expected at their young age to differentiate between healthy risk-taking and hazards that could lead to serious injury or death. A toddler could consider a balance beam elevated at 6 inches to be a risk, but a 12-year-old would have no perception of risk at all. However, a balance beam installed over a hard concrete surface or within a few feet of a concrete seat wall is a hazard that any child, regardless of age, might not recognize as a problem.

Examples of providing varied acceptable risk levels in a play space include complete access for all children to high sections of the play area; slides with different heights and pitches; multiple types of swings (i.e., buckets, disc, tire, belt, basket, and tent); varied climber types (some solid, and others with holes or openings); balance beams of varying widths and heights; features for differing movements and hanging heights, like monkey bars, overhead spinners, and track rides; diverse sizes and widths of mounds and hill climber assistants; and play decks or perimeter walls at varying heights and sizes. Situations that could cause permanent injury or death can be identified by CPSIs trained (based on national playground standards) to look specifically for potential hazards, the most common of which are head injuries, entrapment, protrusions, and pinching.

Sensory-Focused Play

Play is a process children use to avoid or create the sensory experiences they need to interact effectively with the world. Chapter 5, "Sensory Integration: Why it Matters," provided an in-depth description of the eight main sensory systems that should be addressed in an inclusive[+] play space. We invite you to review them as needed.

There are many exciting ways to integrate sensory play into a play space. One unique approach is to incorporate sensory walls. When designed appropriately, these walls help children explore as many of the eight sensory systems as possible with a single feature. Early attempts at sensory walls focused primarily on sight, sound, and texture by applying different materials, like stucco, tile, rubber, metal, and stone. More recent designs incorporate those strategies but expand them to include lights and sounds; a wider range of textures; changes in elevation and depth for exploration of balance (vestibular); large spring-loaded buttons and handles to encourage pushing and pulling, which address proprioception; and materials that hold or reflect varying amounts of heat and cold (interoception).

When designing for younger children (2–5 years old), an exploratory sensory wall should focus more on simple motor experiences, modest elevation change (a couple of feet or meters), simple sounds, and exploration of textures and colors. To note, all the suggestions in the preceding diversity section also apply to a sensory wall. Sensory walls for older children should have a greater focus on more complex gross-motor skills that encourage the exploration of body awareness and balance. This focus can be accomplished through ample pushing, pulling, hanging, and jumping activities. They are most effective when coupled with various textures, colors, and lights. Electronic and mechanical interactive games, like Simon Says, rain sticks, push buttons and switches with integrated lights and sounds, pull chords, hand-spinner games, and abacus racks, are a few examples of items that have been incorporated into sensory walls. Materials that can be used for texture, heat, and visual interest include, among others, polished mirror balls, artificial turf, rubber surfacing, concrete, powder-coated metal, stone, stucco, seashells, hard plastics, outdoor fabrics, wood, bamboo, ceramic tile, and glass tile.

Sensory walks or paths are another option to provide focused sensory experiences. At their basics, sensory walks are a series of instructive steps for a child to follow. Each step represents a specific motion, movement, or sensory experience. A sensory walk might include cues, such as footprints arranged to hop, jump, or leap between. Icons inviting children to stop and spin around, clap their hands, or touch their toes are other sensory cues that can be painted or etched onto walkways. A sensory walk designed for an elementary school in Lathrop, California, incorporates stops along the circular path for twirling, hopping, tiptoeing, skipping, breathing, gazing around, walking with arms out, and other motor movements. The walk also includes stop locations for self-regulation purposes. The walk circles back on itself, so children can continue around the walk until they are ready for another activity. A sensory path is a walkway constructed of various surfacing materials, such as pebbles embedded into concrete, mulch, gravel, bricks, and the like. It is most effective when it is an ancillary, rather than main, pathway because some children will find this an aversive experience, and their desire to avoid traversing over it must be respected. In addition, lest we forget, water- and sand-play systems provide often-mesmerizing multisensory experiences, such as varied textures, temperatures, light refraction patterns, and sounds.

Outdoor musical equipment is another fun approach to creating sensory integrated inclusive[+] play spaces. In recent years, the availability of this equipment has increased, as has the variety of options. In addition to their obvious auditory play value, musical play provides multisensory body awareness and visual, tactile, and auditory play value. At the Seattle Washington Children's PlayGarden, a series of musical instruments flank an easily accessible walkway. Children are encouraged to interact with the colorful and melodic devices from seated or standing positions, using their hands or legs, mallets, or other found objects to create the music of their choice independently or with others.

As a final note, one critical sensory system often overlooked during play space design is interoception (internal regulation). Designing for interoception includes providing ample and varied seating options and shade and water play for body cooling; limiting allergens (refer to previous sections regarding the plant allergen scale); avoiding volatile organic compounds and pollutants in the play space to reduce the risk of allergic reactions; offering food options and planning for dedicated areas to eat, barbeque, or picnic; supplying adequate numbers of accessible drinking fountains and water-bottle filling stations; and providing restrooms with child- and adult-size changing tables nearby.

There are a few things to keep in mind when choosing the best musical equipment for a play space. Foremost, picking equipment usable from both seated and standing positions is crucial. In addition, be sure that some or much of the equipment does not require mallets, tools, or paddles to elicit sound. This allows everyone, regardless of grasping ability or preference, to make music. If mallets or paddles are necessary, larger handles are easier to use. Much of the musical equipment commercially available is fairly susceptible to vandalism. Dance chime products are a good example of how strong and difficult-to-vandalize musical equipment can meet multiple sensory needs (auditory, balance, body awareness, and visual). Try to select robust musical elements that are not made of wood, have few moving parts, and utilize high-strength cables and connections for mallets and similar striking tools. Musical elements mounted to the ground surface with bolts so they can be easily replaced if needed are preferable to mount-in-place installations.

Creative Play

In some capacity, all types of play share the common feature of creativity. Creative play supports learning and social-emotional skills (Fehr & Russ, 2016). Creative play comprises (but is not limited to) explorative, loose parts, dramatic, and themed play.

- Explorative play involves engaging in play activities that do not lose their intrigue. Here, loose parts and nature play may be most intriguing because there is nothing constant about nature; it is always changing.
- Loose parts play items allow children to explore cause-and-effect relationships and methods of manipulating their environment. It can be based on natural items, such as tree cookies or buckets for sand, water, and mud play and bins filled with various sizes of balls.
- Dramatic play provides children ample opportunity to reenact and repeat what they see and hear in their daily lives. Open-ended play features, like playhouses and grassy areas to create imaginary worlds, provide the foundation for dramatic play. The Family Adventure Garden in the San Antonio (Texas) Botanical Garden has a mini-neighborhood of charming little playhouses that beckon dramatic play.
- Community interest and support often drive themed play. We caution you to avoid directing play with overtheming, such as an entire play space focused on animals. Instead, think about also including various animal habitats in the play space, like cozy dens, elevated spaces, and water.

Intergenerational Play

Intergenerational family play is most effectively accomplished through family leisure events that are "unique, shared, interactive, purposive, challenging and requiring sacrifice" (Hebblethwaite & Norris, 2011, p. 123). The challenge with planning for intergenerational play is the differential between each age group's abilities and interests. Including activities in a play space that will engage all ages with each other for any length of time may be difficult. However, given that enough activities exist, multiple generations can spend meaningful time together. Each age group will enjoy some activities more than others.

Older adults may like to go on walks around the play space with their age peers and/or grandchildren and use outdoor fitness equipment on the fringes of the play area. They may gravitate toward working in raised garden or flower beds; playing low-intensity games like bocce ball, corn hole, or horseshoes; picnicking in the play area; or playing board games at tables with chess, checkers, or other game inserts. Older adults may also enjoy sharing storybook readings in small nooks and corners or at raised platforms.

Adolescents may enjoy a mix of active and passive activities, like basketball-shooting games or other court sports, catch ball, skateboarding, pump-track riding, parkour, obstacle courses, challenge games, socializing, and listening to or mixing music with outdoor DJ stations explicitly designed for outdoor recreational spaces. Children may want to explore landscape areas around a play space, play on play equipment or naturalized features, use life-size game boards, play sports, fly kites and drones, and find other creative ways to play.

The beauty is that all these activities can be done together without regard to generational bias—if the right facilities are in place to allow varying levels of engagement. Plan for uninhibited access and then for a range between simple use and highly active, heavy use, and everyone can enjoy participating. The result of everyone being able to participate is that they stay longer and enjoy the interaction with others when they are outside!

Nature-Based Play

Including natural elements provides an educational experience that nurtures hands-on learning and exploration that seldom exists in traditional play spaces. *Several years ago, I (Chad) watched my two young boys get very excited when it began to rain. With little convincing from the boys, my wife happily let them put on rain jackets and boots to explore the wet, new world that appeared so different to them than it had been just a few minutes before. They spent the afternoon chasing leaves and dandelions floating down the street in gutters full of water. They splashed each other, stomped in puddles, and caught and gawked at the snails and worms that emerged, seeking refuge from the saturated landscape. It was joyful to watch them explore what only nature could provide.*

Loose parts play is an intrinsic element of nature that provides a sustained level of diverse and interesting things with which to tinker. We might go so far as to proclaim that a child has not experienced life fully until they have witnessed the mesmerizing movement of maple samaras falling like helicopters from the sky, picked them up, and thrown them back up into the air; stomped in a puddle with no regard to anything but making a splash; or built an obstacle course out of objects found in nature. These are the types of experiences that add depth to the play experience.

We recognize that in formal and dedicated urban spaces, trees and plants might be viewed as messy or unkempt. However, inclusive[+] play spaces are replete with natural loose play elements. A balance between order and mess can be met by providing—but not overdoing—an array of loose-part-creating plants while addressing any maintenance restrictions that may exist. Sometimes, there are conflicts between choices. It will be at the designer's discretion to determine which plant characteristics (e.g., fruiting bodies, leaves and sticks, and flowers and petals) are most important for the project (in the case of inclusive⁺ designs, allergen levels versus play value is paramount).

Fruiting Bodies

The fruiting bodies of plants are amazing elements for dramatic and exploratory play. Some of the many types of plant fruits appropriate for play areas include berries, drupes, catkins, seed pods or capsules, achenes, samaras, nuts, and cones. Here are a few examples of plants that produce these types of fruits yet have mostly dry, manageable litter. However, please tap into your regional options:

- Berries and fruits: India hawthorne, strawberry tree, Chinese pistache, heavenly bamboo, Tilia species, and junipers
- Catkins: alder and birch trees
- Seed pods: honeylocust, catalpa, redbud, desert willow, palo verde, chitalpa, and mimosa trees
- Achenes: sycamore, buckeye, and sweet-gum tree; dandelions; sunflowers
- Samaras: maple, ash, and elm trees
- Nuts: oak, hornbeam, and horse chestnut trees
- Cones: pine, spruce, fir, redwood, cypress, and hemlock trees and shrubs

Leaves and Sticks

In addition to fruiting bodies, some plants offer excellent play value through other aspects, such as interesting leaf sizes, shapes, colors, and the production of litter, like needles and twigs. All these components can inspire dramatic and creative play, such as spontaneous swashbuckling sword fights, fall leaf-drop mazes, leaf crown crafts, and mini-military stick forts. Here are a few examples of plants that can produce these types of opportunities, but please tap into your regional options:

- Interesting leaves: catalpa, sycamore, tulip tree; maple, oak, horse chestnut, and mimosa trees; African iris, phormium, red-hot poker, juniper, decorative grasses, lamb's ears, rosemary, cape's rush, spineless aloes, and horsetails
- Needles: pine, spruce, fir, redwood, and hemlock trees and shrubs
- Sticks and twigs: ash, elm, bamboo, willow, and dogwood

Flowers and Petals

Other plants offer play value through their flowers' vibrant colors, fragrances, and shapes. Flowers can captivate the attention of young and old and are great catalysts for exploratory and dramatic play. Children greatly enjoy collecting and delivering flowers. This should be considered an acceptable element of play and encouraged wherever possible. Here are a few examples of interesting flowers that can produce these types of opportunities, but please tap into your regional options: red-hot poker, lavender, African iris, sage, bleeding heart plant, crocus, California poppy, yarrow, dandelions, sunflowers, society garlic, kangaroo paw, hardy hibiscus, rockrose, lilac, rose mallow, butterfly bush, echinacea, snake grass, sedge species, periwinkle, Japanese snowball bush (viburnum), and fountain grasses.

This discussion barely scratches the surface of the many play opportunities plants offer children and adults. Full-blown expeditions, filled with treasure and adventure, happen in play environments every day all over the world. Hopefully, this information will encourage infusion of plants into these environments and provide great potential for successful creative play.

Trauma-Responsive Play

Children who have or are experiencing trauma in their lives need opportunities to play. It is an essential part of what they need to help them heal, grow, and develop. Through intensive collaboration with health care professionals, we can support trauma-responsive play with the following design considerations:

- Create opportunities to rebuild a sense of control, comfort, and empowerment. Creating or changing the environment alone is not enough. The broader goal is for the built environment to support any type of therapeutic programs, such as sensory diets or lifestyles and welcoming service animals.
- Remove adverse environmental stresses when possible.
- Provide security in multiple ways, such as lighting, no dead-end paths or closed structures, and clear site lines within the play space to provide safety.
- Design clean, easy-to-understand spaces that do not elicit stress or a sense of confusion.
- Create separation spaces to which those in distress can retreat.
- Reinforce personal agency.
- Encourage personal identity through play elements that encourage self-discovery.
- Provide areas of refuge and "onlooking" that feel safe and comforting.
- Above all else, diversify the space to provide opportunities for multiple situational needs.

Figures 7.6–7.8 show examples of how well-planned and designed play elements can address the various social considerations integral to inclusive[+] play space design. We also include a template to help you plan inclusive[+] play spaces.

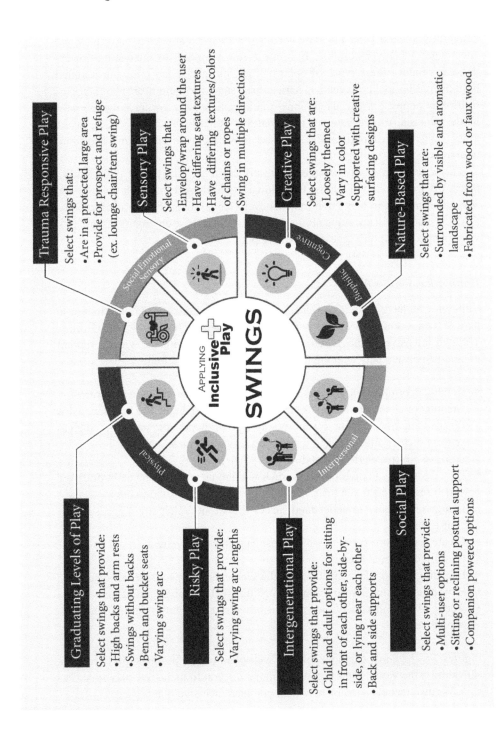

Trauma Responsive Play

Select swings that:
- Are in a protected large area
- Provide for prospect and refuge (ex. lounge chair/tent swing)

Sensory Play

Select swings that:
- Envelop/wrap around the user
- Have differing seat textures
- Have differing textures/colors of chains or ropes
- Swing in multiple direction

Creative Play

Select swings that are:
- Loosely themed
- Vary in color
- Supported with creative surfacing designs

Nature-Based Play

Select swings that are:
- Surrounded by visible and aromatic landscape
- Fabricated from wood or faux wood

Graduating Levels of Play

Select swings that provide:
- High backs and arm rests
- Swings without backs
- Bench and bucket seats
- Varying swing arc

Risky Play

Select swings that provide:
- Varying swing arc lengths

Intergenerational Play

Select swings that provide:
- Child and adult options for sitting in front of each other, side-by-side, or lying near each other
- Back and side supports

Social Play

Select swings that provide:
- Multi-user options
- Sitting or reclining postural support
- Companion powered options

APPLYING Inclusive Play

SWINGS

Social Emotional
Sensory
Cognitive
Biophilic
Interpersonal
Physical

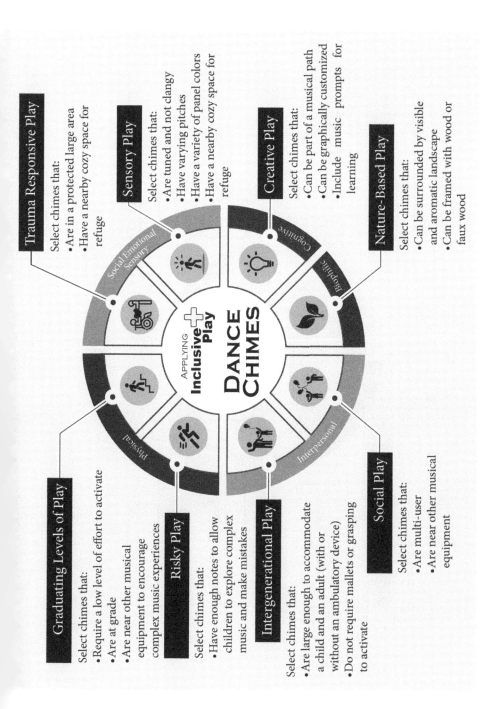

Trauma Responsive Play

Select chimes that:
• Are in a protected large area
• Have a nearby cozy space for refuge

Sensory Play

Select chimes that:
• Are tuned and not clangy
• Have varying pitches
• Have a variety of panel colors
• Have a nearby cozy space for refuge

Creative Play

Select chimes that:
• Can be part of a musical path
• Can be graphically customized
• Include music prompts for learning

Nature-Based Play

Select chimes that:
• Can be surrounded by visible and aromatic landscape
• Can be framed with wood or faux wood

Graduating Levels of Play

Select chimes that:
• Require a low level of effort to activate
• Are at grade
• Are near other musical equipment to encourage complex music experiences

Risky Play

Select chimes that:
• Have enough notes to allow children to explore complex music and make mistakes

Intergenerational Play

Select chimes that:
• Are large enough to accommodate a child and an adult (with or without an ambulatory device)
• Do not require mallets or grasping to activate

Social Play

Select chimes that:
• Are multi-user
• Are near other musical equipment

FIGURE 7.7 Social considerations for an Inclusive⁺ Play Space: Dance chimes.

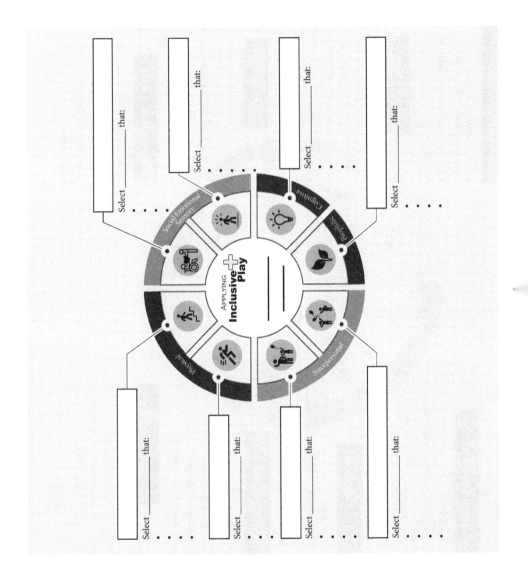

Final Thoughts

Inclusive[+] play space design extends far beyond the play elements and equipment selected. Considerations for how all types of play can flourish are just as important as what the play space contains. In essence, inclusive[+] play space design takes into account the vital relationship between children and the play space environment. Layered on top of the relationship between the child and their space is that inclusive[+] play spaces support them in doing what they want and need to do to nourish their bodies, minds, and emotions. An inclusive[+] play space embraces the notion that all children and their families can be their best selves when we create spaces that welcome them—on their terms—to play as they need to play. This chapter provides the scaffolding for you to design inclusive[+] play spaces that meet the children where they are and help them become who they want to be.

BOX 7.1   CASE STUDY: MAY NISSAN PLAYGROUND (FIGURES 7.9–7.14)

Project Information:

Name
May Nissen Playground
Designer
O'Dell Engineering
Location
Pleasanton, CA
Size
7,610 m² or 1.88 acres
Year Built
2019
Age Group(s)
2–5 years, 5–12 years, and intergenerational

Description:

The May Nissen Playground is a 1.88-acre play space in Livermore, California, adjacent to a local library and aquatic facility. This 100% socially inclusive play space features areas for outdoor reading and theatrical, dramatic, and creative play to complement the library operations. It also features multiple play areas, adaptive outdoor exercise equipment, and a new gender-neutral inclusive restroom facility. Theming for the May Nissen Playground draws inspiration from classic fairy tales like "Jack and the Beanstalk."

The play space was intentionally designed out of scale, with oversized leaf-shaped art, large grade changes, and gigantic overhead flower structures to create the illusion of being small in a big space. Other features, such as cozy social spaces, an interactive performance stage, colorful pavement treatments, and woodland-like features, transport children wherever their imagination might take them. The community helped champion this project and was heavily involved in the design.

(Continued)

Websites:

- https://www.larpd.org/maps/location/MayNissenPark
- https://www.playlsi.com/en/commercial-playground-equipment/playgrounds/may-nissen-park/

Traditional Inclusive Features	Inclusive⁺ Features
• Accessible path of travel • Accessible structures • Accessible swings • PIP rubber surfacing • Accessible slides • Accessible climbers • Completely fenced perimeter for safety	• Having no ramps limits the required physical effort to navigate the play space • Nature-based theme to enhance exploratory play options • Double-wide roller slide to encourage social play • Multiple cozy spaces for self-regulation and restoration • Multisensory integrated story nook with stage and interactive story and music equipment • Life-size interactive game boards to encourage social interaction • Roll-under capacity in raised water and sand play that encourages social interaction and sensory play • Accessible gender-neutral restroom • Integrated landscape and natural elements to encourage loose parts play • Integrated grade changes that provide movement challenges • Overarching play approach focuses on social integration • Intergenerational play options include adaptive exercise equipment to bring families and caregivers together in an outdoor environment • Play-related dramatic art features encourage imaginative play and interaction • Integrated companion seating benches and tables for comfort and socialization • Integrated and natural shade options to help with temperature and internal regulation

Remarks:

This project is a shining example of what an inclusive⁺ play space can and should be. It can be a magical place that fosters creative play, it transcends accessibility to include diversity in play and rest opportunities, integrates all eight sensory systems, and promotes socially interactive play without the need for it to be prescribed. Children find their own adventures in this play space. With 207 inclusive-play opportunities throughout the play space, there is no shortage of fun to be discovered or created. These opportunities are spread across the spectrum of inclusive needs, including features that provide cognitive, sensory (basic five senses), physical, interoceptive, proprioceptive, vestibular, and social enrichment.

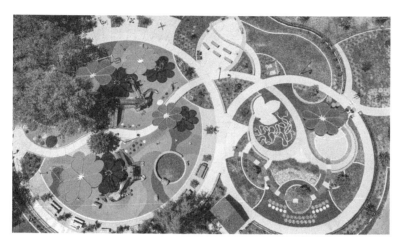

FIGURE 7.9   Bird's eye view. Credit- Landscape Structures Inc.

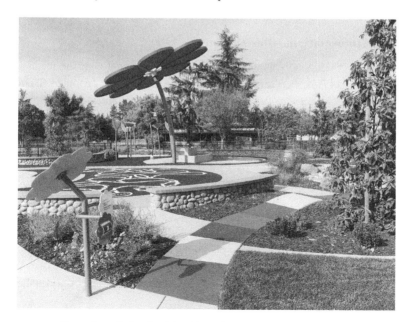

FIGURE 7.10   Game board. Credit- O'Dell Engineering.

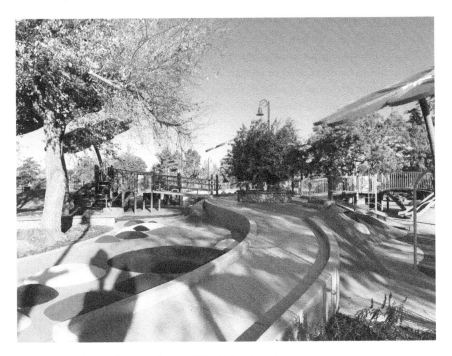

FIGURE 7.11   Ramped entry. Credit- O'Dell Engineering.

BOX 7.2   CASE STUDY: EMPOWERMENT PARK (FIGURES 7.12–7.14)

Project Information:

Name
EmPOWERment Park

Designer
O'DellEngineering, Amy Wagenfeld | Design, Keith Christensen

Location
Sacramento, CA

Size
5,260 m² or 1.3 acres

Year Built
2023

Age Group(s)
2–5 and 5–12 years, intergenerational

Description:

EmPOWERment Park is designed with socially inclusive principles to be a place where people of all abilities and ages can gather to play and recreate. The park features an energy/electricity theme to honor and show appreciation to the Sacramento Municipal Utility District for donating the land that made it possible. The park includes educational features highlighting the many ways power is provided daily to the community. Sustainability was a significant focus during the design process, with the inclusion of features promoting wise stewardship of resources. The space was carefully planned to address myriad childhood development needs while providing universal access, socially inclusive and sensory-integrated opportunities,

(Continued)

(Continued)

and intergenerational play options. The community was heavily engaged in the design process.
Public outreach included conversations with community members at festivals, events, and schools;
a self-guided tour of play, addressing all the needs
of people and play; team-building activities; and a
"test-it-out" meeting, where the public could walk
through and experience a pop-up demonstration of
the future park.

Website:

* https://www.sacparksfoundation.org/empowerment-park

Traditional Inclusive Features	Inclusive⁺ Features
• Accessible path of travel • Accessible structures • Accessible swings • PIP rubber surfacing • Accessible slides • Accessible climbers • Completely fenced perimeter for safety	• Having limited ramps reduces the required physical effort to navigate the play space • Highest elevations are accessible to everyone and are the largest gathering spaces in the play space • Double-wide slides to encourage social play • Transition stations at the bottom of the slides • Multiple cozy spaces for self-regulation and restoration • Multisystem sensory walls to experience all the sensory systems in early childhood and child age-group areas • Self-cleaning, inclusive restroom with adult-size changing table and crane lift • Integrated landscape and natural elements to encourage loose parts play • Integrated grade changes that provide movement challenges • Overarching play approach focused on social integration • Intergenerational play options to bring families and caregivers together • Companion seating benches and tables for comfort and socialization • Themed zones and path hierarchy for ease of understanding

(*Continued*)

(Continued)

Traditional Inclusive Features	Inclusive⁺ Features
	• Accessible parking stalls maximize access to the play space • Integrated and natural shade options to help with temperature regulation • Adaptive basketball-hoop game system and customized plaza games encourage social play • Accessible community-garden raised planter beds

Remarks:

This play space does a great job of implementing recent research into the project. One example is the oversized decks at the top of the 5- to 12-year-old play area. Many of the play area's fun and exciting elements are located at the highest point, where there is plenty of room for children to congregate and socialize. The play's features were thought through in great detail to ensure everyone could use them. These features include panels with handles large enough to use without grasping, musical equipment with lever activators and not mallets, Braille and raised-letter signs and instructions, double-wide ramps for efficient movement, and color-coordinated play areas for simple identification.

The looped walkway is a simple travel way to start and stop at the same location, providing essential cognitive simplicity. The electronics theme is not overdone but gives just enough context to aid in educating about and understanding the power sources in the region. Even the sensory walls, which tactfully educate about power and energy, were carefully designed for the appropriate age groups. The younger age group's wall focuses more on fine-motor skills and the exploration of touch, sight, and sound senses through varied imagery, colors, textures, and small grasping-type activities. The older group's wall focuses more on combining all sensory groups, with a heavier emphasis on the vestibular and proprioceptive systems through running, climbing, pulling, pushing, and interactive light and sound games. The increasing challenge and difficulty levels of the sensory walls and other equipment give children a wide variety of options and keep their interest.

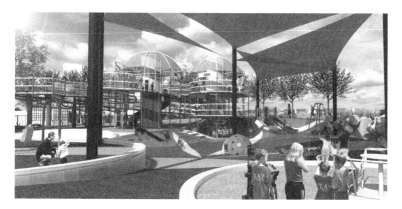

FIGURE 7.12   Big play structure. Credit- O'Dell Engineering.

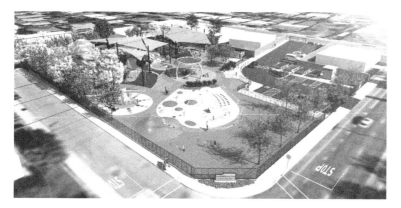

FIGURE 7.13   Bird's eye over Bell Street. Credit- O'Dell Engineering.

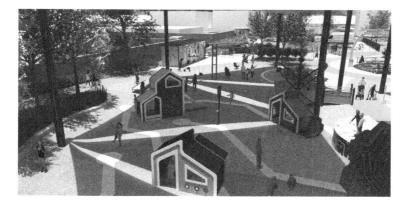

FIGURE 7.14   Circuit city. Credit- O'Dell Engineering.

References

Brown, D. M., Ross, T., Leo, J., Buliung, R. N., Shirazipour, C. H., Latimer-Cheung, A. E., & Arbour-Nicitopoulos, K. P. (2021). A scoping review of evidence-informed recommendations for designing inclusive playgrounds. *Frontiers in Rehabilitation Sciences, 2,* Article 664595. https://doi.org/10.3389/fresc.2021.664595

Brussoni, M., Olsen, L. L., Pike, I., & Sleet, D. A. (2012). Risky play and children's safety: Balancing priorities for optimal child development. *International Journal of Environmental Research and Public Health, 9*(9), 3134–3148. https://doi.org/10.3390/ijerph9093134

Children and Nature Network. (2020). *The equigenic effect: How nature access can level the playing field for children.* https://www.childrenandnature.org/resources/the-equigenic-effect-how-nature-access-can-level-the-playing-field-for-children

Coates, J. K., & Pimlott-Wilson, H. (2019). Learning while playing: Children's forest school experiences in the UK. *British Educational Research Journal, 45*(1), 21–40. https://doi.org/10.1002/berj.3491

Farroni, T., Csibra, G., Simion, F., & Johnson, M. H. (2002). Eye contact detection in humans from birth. *Proceedings of the National Academy of Sciences, 99*(14), 9602–9605. https://doi.org/10.1073/pnas.152159999

Fehr, K. K., & Russ, S. W. (2016). Pretend play and creativity in preschool-age children: Associations and brief intervention. *Psychology of Aesthetics, Creativity, and the Arts, 10*(3), 296–308. https://doi.org/10.1037/aca0000054

Gil, J. D., Ewerling, F., Ferreira, L. Z., & Barros, A. J. (2020). Early childhood suspected developmental delay in 63 low-and middle-income countries: Large within-and between-country inequalities documented using national health surveys. *Journal of Global Health, 10*(1), Article 010427. https://doi.org/10.7189/jogh.10.010427

Gleave, J. (2008). *Risk and play.* https://www.springzaad.nl/wp-content/uploads/2020/04/risk_and_play-a_literature_review.pdf

Hebblethwaite, S., & Norris, J. (2011). Expressions of generativity through family leisure: Experiences of grandparents and adult grandchildren. *Family Relations, 60,* 121–133. https://doi.org/10.1111/j.1741-3729.2010.00637.x

Jenkins, G. R., Yuen, H. K., Rose, E. J., Maher, A. I., Gregory, K. C., & Cotton, M. E. (2015). Disparities in quality of park play spaces between two cities with diverse income and race/ethnicity composition: A pilot study. *International Journal of Environmental Research and Public Health, 12*(7), 8009–8022. https://doi.org/10.3390/ijerph120708009

Jongerius, C., Hessels, R. S., Romijn, J. A., Smets, E. M., & Hillen, M. A. (2020). The measurement of eye contact in human interactions: A scoping review. *Journal of Nonverbal Behavior, 44,* 363–389. https://doi.org/10.1007/s10919-020-00333-3

Lifter, K., Sulzer-Azaroff, B., Anderson, S. R., & Cowdery, G. E. (1993). Teaching play activities to preschool children with disabilities: The importance of developmental considerations. *Journal of Early Intervention, 17*(2), 139–159. https://doi.org/10.1177/105381519301700206

Mitchell, R., Shortt, N., Richardson, E., & Pearce, J. (2014). Is access to green space associated with smaller socio-economic inequalities in mental wellbeing among urban dwellers across Europe? *European Journal of Public Health, 24*(suppl_2), 15–16. https://doi.org/10.1093/eurpub/cku151.022

Mitchell, R. J., Richardson, E. A., Shortt, N. K., & Pearce, J. R. (2015). Neighborhood environments and socioeconomic inequalities in mental well-being. *American Journal of Preventive Medicine, 49*(1), 80–84. https://doi.org/10.1016/j.amepre.2015.01.017

Murniyati, B., & Wardhani, J. D. (2023). Economic token techniques as an effort to increase the independence of children aged 4-5 years. *Early Childhood Research Journal (ECRJ)*, *5*(2), 29–43. https://doi.org/10.23917/ecrj.v5i2.20834

National Public Radio. (2013). *NPR reports on accessible playgrounds & maps more than 1,300 around the U.S.* https://www.npr.org/about-npr/216127699/npr-reports-on-accessible-playgrounds-maps-more-than-1-300-around-the-u-s

Niedźwiecka, A. (2020). Look me in the eyes: Mechanisms underlying the eye contact effect. *Child Development Perspectives, 14*(2), 78–82. https://doi.org/10.1111/cdep.12361

Siu, K. W. M., Wong, Y. L., & Lam, M. S. (2017). Inclusive play in urban cities: A pilot study of the inclusive playgrounds in Hong Kong. *Procedia Engineering, 198*, 169–175. https://doi.org/10.1016/j.proeng.2017.07.080

Smythe, T., Zuurmond, M., Tann, C. J., Gladstone, M., & Kuper, H. (2021). Early intervention for children with developmental disabilities in low and middle-income countries: The case for action. *International Health, 13*(3), 222–231. https://doi.org/10.1093/inthealth/ihaa044

State of California Natural Resources Agency. (2023). *Application guide. Land and water conservation fund*. Department of Parks and Recreation Office of Grants and Local Services. https://www.parks.ca.gov/pages/1008/files/LWCF%20Application%20Guide%202023%20Final%20Draft%2011.22.22.pdf

Sunarty, K., & Dirawan Darma, G. (2015). Development parenting model to increase the independence of children. *International Education Studies, 8*(10), 1–213. https://doi.org/10.5539/ies.8n10p107

Tai, L. (2022). *Letting play bloom: Designing nature-based risky play for children*. Temple University Press.

Van Melik, R., & Althuizen, N. (2022). Inclusive play policies: Disabled children and their access to Dutch playgrounds. *Journal of Economic and Human Geography, 113*(2), 117–130. https://doi.org/10.1111/tesg.12457

Wenger, I., Schulze, C., Lundström, U., & Prellwitz, M. (2021). Children's perceptions of playing on inclusive playgrounds: A qualitative study. *Scandinavian Journal of Occupational Therapy, 28*(2), 136–146. https://doi.org/10.1080/11038128.2020.1810768

AFTERWORD

We end where we started, inviting you, the reader, to consider the extraordinary value of being outside and the importance of inclusive outdoor play spaces. With an ever-increasing body of research validating the global health benefits that can happen when we are outside, it makes sense that there must be equitable access for everyone to have opportunities to be outside. Being in nature helps children feel calmer, more resilient, and more focused. Nature can be a catalyst for learning to play together; learning happens in real time when outside. Children who have opportunities to be outside during their school day return to the classroom more focused and ready to learn. Playing outside can—and does—make children stronger and helps reduce obesity. Playing should be fun. Playing should be available for anyone who wants to give it a go.

Play is the most important job of childhood, and no child deserves to be denied access to play—be it at home, at school, or in the community. Recall Carina, the little girl who longed to play with her peers. Sadly, no matter what play space she and her mom visited, none accommodated her needs. In the end, she would always leave yet another play space without having experienced the joys of exploring or climbing or the spontaneous and creative interaction she desired with her peers. This is unjust.

Let's rewind the tape on this: Take a step back and think about how you—the designer, therapist, educator, or caregiver—can be the catalyst to effect change for the better. This change must occur so the Carinas of the world (and their caregivers) can confidently go to a play space knowing the children will have equal opportunities to play, whether or not their challenges are visible. The increasingly robust evidence that connecting with nature supports physical, sensory, social-emotional, and cognitive development establishes the rationale to convince any doubting or reluctant clients, funders, and other decision-makers that outdoor play spaces matter for the health and wellness of children and their adults. This extends to all play spaces, not just inclusive ones. Children need to be outside, preferably at least 30 minutes every day, but more is better. An inclusive play space—ideally located near their home, easily accessible via public transportation, or on their school grounds— enables children to do just that.

A *New York Times* article profiling civil rights activist Michael Skolnik shared, "The truth is we need all kinds of people playing together in this sandbox" (Feuer, 2015, para. 28). No matter one's abilities and skills, age, gender, socioeconomic or sociogeographic status, race, or cultural identity, everyone needs the opportunity to play, learn, and experience a sandbox. This sandbox could be an actual sandbox designed to meet the needs of children with various challenges. It also could be a metaphor loudly reminding us that everyone needs to be able to play.

We need today's children to grow up healthy and ready to take on whatever challenges they may face. We need the adults in their lives to feel confident in their choices to let their children play on their own terms, no matter who they are. We need children to experience risky play to understand the boundaries of their bodies. And we must have future generations of children who need not suffer the indignity of being unable to play at a play space identified as "accessible" or "inclusive." We invite you to take on the exciting challenge of designing inclusive+ play spaces that inspire and delight children because, at heart, we are all children who yearn to play and experience joy and happiness.

Reference

Feuer, A. (2015, November 20). Michael Skolnik taps his social network to fight for civil rights. New York Times. https://www.nytimes.com/2015/11/22/nyregion/michael-skolnik-political-director-for-russell-simmons-fights-for-civil-rights.html

INDEX

Note: **Bold** page numbers refer to tables and *italic* page numbers refer to figures.

For Product Safety Concerns and Information please contact our EU
representative GPSR@taylorandfrancis.com Taylor & Francis Verlag GmbH,
Kaufingerstraße 24, 80331 München, Germany

Printed and bound by CPI Group (UK) Ltd, Croydon, CR0 4YY
01/05/2025
01858504-0001